ABORTION FREE

YOUR MANUAL *for* BUILDING *a* PRO-LIFE AMERICA ONE COMMUNITY *at a* TIME

TROY NEWMAN &

CHERYL SULLENGER

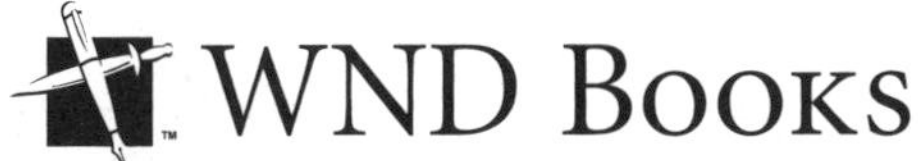

ABORTION FREE

Book designed by Mark Karis
Cover illustration by Michael Di Pietro—inspired by illustration by Katie Edwards.

WND Books are distributed to the trade by:
Midpoint Trade Books, 27 West 20th Street, Suite 1102, New York, New York 10011

WND Books are available at special discounts for bulk purchases.
WND Books, Inc., also publishes books in electronic formats.
For more information call (541) 474-1776 or visit www.wndbooks.com.

First Edition
Paperback ISBN: 978-1-936488-22-3 eBook ISBN: 978-1-936488-23-0

Library of Congress Cataloging-in-Publication Data
Newman, Troy, 1966-
Abortion free : your manual for building a pro-life America one community at a time / by Troy Newman and Cheryl Sullenger. -- First edition.
pages cm
ISBN 978-1-936488-22-3 (paperback) -- ISBN 978-1-936488-23-0 (e-book)
1. Pro-life movement--United States. 2. Abortion services--United States. 3. Abortion--Religious aspects--Christianity. 4. Abortion--Moral and ethical aspects--United States. I. Sullenger, Cheryl. II. Title.
HQ767.5.U5N47 2014
363.460973--dc23
2014012698

Printed in the United States of America
10 9 8 7 6 5 4 3 2 1

We dedicate this book to our families, particularly our spouses, Mellissa Newman-Mariotti and Randall Sullenger, who have sacrificed much so we could pursue—often obsessively—the call that God placed on our hearts to defend the defenseless, speak for the voiceless, and expose the unfruitful works of darkness all with the hope of ending the scourge of abortion in our lifetimes.

CONTENTS

PART 3: NUTS AND BOLTS

FOREWORD

People perish for lack of knowledge. Babies, mothers, and entire communities are perishing from the scourge of abortion. And yet people do not know the truth about abortion. It is the killing of innocent babies, and it inflicts misery upon the lives of vulnerable women. I for one hid the truth regarding my abortions for many years, until I heard the truth about abortion and found freedom from guilt and shame. That is why Troy Newman and Cheryl Sullenger invited me to write this foreword; I appreciate the honor of adding my testimony to their journals.

Since 1983 I have delivered the truth about abortion from a public platform. Many know my voice from the work I do as director of African American outreach for Priests for Life where I am also a spokeswoman for The Silent No More Awareness Campaign. I also have received healing from the Priests for Life's Rachael's Vineyard abortion recovery ministry. It is through this work that I met Troy and Cheryl and came to know of their powerful efforts at Operation Rescue (OR) to uncover and dismantle the harmful forces that drive the abortion industry.

The truth of abortion bothers them so much that they have devoted years of research and activism to exposing the stark reality about the licensed-to-kill doctors who are slaughtering our innocent babies. They have spent a collective lifetime not only exposing the horrors of what goes on behind the closed doors of abortion mills but also diligently working to close these killing centers down for good. And they are succeeding.

Their research, awareness crusades, and direct intervention continues to break down the once impenetrable barriers between the unsuspecting general public and the killing of the unborn. They reveal the secret wealth of the abortion mills that are paid to commit the genocide.

Troy and Cheryl are not alone in this quest; truly there are hundreds of thousands of foot soldiers who give their all every day to defend the sanctity of life. We commend every warrior as we support Troy and Cheryl in their work laboring on the frontlines of the war as pillars in the vanguard in the battle for life. Where once people had no idea about the horrors of abortion, now they do.

Abortion Free is not a suggestion. *Abortion Free* is a promise that there will be an end to the scourge of abortion. Thanks in a large part to the efforts of Operation Rescue, cofounded by Newman and Sullenger, our society is moving in the direction of fewer and safer abortions.

My uncle Dr. Martin Luther King, Jr., often spoke about the sanctity of all life. He preached compassion against "man's inhumanity to man." He once said that "injustice anywhere is a threat to justice everywhere." Thanks to OR and now this new book *Abortion Free,* the dream has wings. There are now compelling testimonies from the front lines in the battle for life, as well as the detailed how-to steps to exposing the repugnant practices inside the killing centers. For the motivated and the purpose-driven souls who want to end the gruesome practice of killing babies and maiming mothers, *Abortion Free* answers not only the question How do you close abortion clinics. Indeed it also includes in plain language the tested and vetted steps to closing these killing centers and making America abortion free. This is twenty-first-century divine intervention.

Finally, as a minister of the Gospel of Jesus Christ, Who is absolutely "the Way, the Truth and the Life," I believe that we must be grateful that Troy and Cheryl understand the connection between the gospel truth and the gospel of life. In this practical how-to guide to ending the scourge of abortion, I believe we will discover a vital weapon in a war that is not only winnable but one that is being won. Let us march onward towards the freedom in the liberty awaiting us in this compelling volume.

—**DR. ALVEDA KING**

Dr. Alveda C. King is the Director of African American Outreach for Priests for Life, and Founder of Alveda King Ministries. She is a mother, grandmother, Gospel minister, singer, songwriter, producer, and author.

PREFACE

A lot has changed since Operation Rescue first burst into national headlines in 1988, with mass arrests at abortion clinics in Atlanta, Georgia, during the Democratic Convention, and later in 1991, during the Summer of Mercy protests in Wichita, Kansas. At that time, Operation Rescue oversaw the largest peaceful civil disobedience movement in American history.

Changes in culture and the advent of the Freedom of Access to Clinic Entrances Act of 1994, which made abortion clinic blockades a federal crime with long jail terms even for a first offense, forced Operation Rescue to develop new tactics to close abortion clinics. The peaceful sit-ins, known as Rescues, would close an abortion clinic for a few hours or maybe a full day, but they would result in lengthy court hearings, fines, and often jail time. Today, Operation Rescue employs new tactics that are closing abortion clinics permanently.

That change has resulted from Troy Newman's taking the helm of Operation Rescue in 1999 and remaking it into the successful cutting-edge and nationally recognized organization it is today. He and this book's coauthor, Cheryl Sullenger, began developing these tactics in San Diego, California; honed them in Wichita, Kansas; and perfected them in projects around the nation. Their new tactics have been at least partially responsible for the multiplying number of abortion clinic closures in recent years.

Troy was born to a single mother in Anchorage, Alaska, in 1966 and was adopted by a family in San Diego, California, where he grew up enjoying the sun and surfer culture.

His life took a turn when he dedicated it to Jesus Christ in early adulthood. He dreamed of becoming a "preacher boy," perhaps one day pastoring a church. In 1991, he married his wife, Mellissa, and settled into family life working in the computer field while studying the Scriptures.

The course of his life would dramatically shift again when God placed upon his heart a burden to save babies from abortion. Troy worked with Cheryl in San Diego during the 1990s, where their combined work helped close eighteen abortion clinics in San Diego County alone over a ten-year time period.

As a result of Troy's pro-life work, he determined to seek out his birth parents to thank them for the gift of life. Troy's quest was successful, and he was reunited with his natural mother and father, who are now actively involved in his life.

Troy understood that to accomplish his dream of an abortion-free America, it would take more than a part-time effort, so he quit his computer job and took a full-time position with Operation Rescue. He moved his growing family to Lake Arrowhead to continue his pro-life work from the headquarters of what was then Operation Rescue of California, later renamed Operation Rescue West and finally just Operation Rescue.

Troy moved Operation Rescue to Wichita, Kansas, in 2002, along with his family, where they continue to live on a small ranch in rural Kansas. Now the father of five homeschooled children, Troy and his active family enjoy horseback riding, hunting, traveling, and physical fitness. Troy holds a second-degree black belt in Tae Kwon Do. With a sharp mind for business, he helps to augment his family's income by buying and selling real estate in his spare time.

Troy is an in-demand pro-life speaker who travels extensively, encouraging activists around the nation. He is an accomplished spokesman for the pro-life cause and has been featured in such notable publications as *Rolling Stone Magazine,* the *Los Angeles Times,* and the *Chicago Tribune.* His quotes have appeared in nearly every major news publication.

Cheryl was born in Marshalltown, Iowa, in the midst of the post–World War II baby boom in 1955. A hunger for truth led her to receive Christ in 1976 while attending college in Des Moines, after Christians conducting door-to-door evangelism shared the gospel with her. Two weeks later, she joined Shiloh Youth Revival Centers, a nationwide network of Christian communal houses that reached out to America's youth during the heyday of the Jesus movement.

Cheryl served briefly as a missionary in Salt Lake City, Utah, before attending Bible school. She graduated in early 1978, at Shiloh's beautiful eighty-eight-acre study center nestled in the foothills of the Cascades outside Eugene, Oregon.

After completing Bible school, Cheryl was sent to staff Shiloh houses in Alaska, where she lived for three years. There, she met and married her husband, Randall, in 1979. Cheryl and her new husband later moved to San Diego, California, where they raised their two daughters.

After a time as a stay-at-home mom, Cheryl became involved in pro-life ministry in 1984, first serving as a volunteer counselor at a crisis pregnancy center, then as an on-site sidewalk counselor outside abortion clinics in Southern California, during which time she helped save approximately twenty-five hundred babies from abortion.

For seven years, Cheryl taught a combined third- and fourth-grade class at a private Christian school in San Diego's East County suburb of Santee. During this time she founded the California Life Coalition, a pro-life group that engaged in sidewalk counseling and other First Amendment outreaches. For years she organized major annual events in San Diego, including Life Chain and outreaches at the heavily attended Earth Day Fair. In addition, she served two years as a publicly elected member of the San Diego Republican Party.

In 2003, Cheryl and her family moved to Wichita, to work with Troy and Operation Rescue. Over the next two years, while fully engaged in Operation Rescue's intensive project in Wichita, she helped her husband overcome decades of alcoholism. Today, Randall is a proud graduate of Hebron Addiction Recovery Program for Men in Bloomington, Indiana. By the grace of God, he has enjoyed nearly a decade of sobriety, thanks in part to Cheryl's steadfast support, and now works as a produce manager for a grocery chain.

Cheryl is also an experienced media spokesperson and a published editorialist who writes extensively concerning life issues. Her articles are regularly published by pro-life/pro-family news sites, and her quotes have appeared in the *New York Times*, on the website of Bloomberg News, and in other major national news publications.

Cheryl and Randall are the delighted grandparents of eight beautiful grandchildren. Cheryl was blessed to have attended the birth of each one. She has a passion for IndyCar Series open-wheeled racing, science fiction, and creative endeavors such as crafting and cake decorating.

Together Troy Newman and Cheryl Sullenger are a formidable team that has transformed what it means to be pro-life activists.

Because of Troy's visionary leadership role, he is the narrator of this book, although Cheryl has done most of the actual writing. The authors chose to present the book this way in order to simplify the narrative for the reader's sake.

Troy and Cheryl owe much to the steadfast support of many who have made this work possible. Rev. Patrick Mahoney, founder and director of the Christian Defense Coalition, has served as a longtime friend and sounding board for many ideas. Dr. Gary Cass, director of DefendChristians.org, has been an invaluable spiritual adviser. We have been blessed with relationships with many excellent pro-life groups that have all aided in some way in advancing our new strategies, including Priests for Life, Life Dynamics Inc., Americans United for Life, Life Legal Defense Foundation, and many more.

The entire Myers family of Kansas are owed a debt for their longtime support and encouragement, but we especially thank Nellie Myers for investing long hours proofreading our manuscript, and her daughter, Deborah, who serves as our primary assistant and is a brilliant researcher.

To those who have faithfully supported the work of Operation Rescue financially and through prayer, we express deep gratitude for sticking with us through the peaks as well as the valleys, and for believing in our work. Without you, the lifesaving efforts of Operation Rescue would not have been able to continue. Our victories, for which we humbly thank God, are yours as well.

PART 1

GETTING STARTED

1

WHEN ABORTION CLINICS CLOSE, LIVES ARE SAVED

If you want to be successful, it's just this simple. Know what you are doing. Love what you are doing. And believe in what you are doing.

—**WILL ROGERS**

Let me start with a confession. I like it—no, I love it—when abortion clinics close. When the news hits that another abortion clinic has shut down or that some abortionist has been stripped of his medical license, my senior policy adviser, coauthor, and friend Cheryl Sullenger and I break out the old standard "Another One Bites the Dust" from the rock band Queen and play what has become our anthem at full volume as our entire office staff celebrates and sings along.

There is reason to observe and rejoice in the demise of an abortion clinic. For more than forty years, America has failed in its experiment with abortion on demand through all nine months of human gestation. It's an experiment that has gone horribly wrong in terms of human suffering. Our morgues have been the tragic "final stop" for the bodies of mothers who were victims of botched abortions, and our landfills have become macabre depositories for the discarded remains of pre-born children that are treated as trash in life and in death.

Just as the sting of alcoholism touches everyone in an alcoholic's life, it is hard to find a person that has not been touched in some way by abortion. Three out of every ten American women will have had at least one abortion by the time they reach forty-five. The pain of abortion runs deep. Moms and dads, brothers and sisters, grandparents and friends all experience a terrible sense of loss when a pre-born baby is taken by the abortion cartel. That anguish forces those who have experienced abortion to rarely talk about it, and some keep the secret even from their closest friends. The stigma attached to abortion today stems from the heartache of those who experience it.

In order to improve the public perception of abortion, the largest abortion provider in the world, Planned Parenthood, began marketing T-shirts emblazoned with the slogan "I had an abortion." In 2004 the shirts sold for fifteen dollars. I'm sure Planned Parenthood expected to sell them by the millions, but I have never, ever seen a woman wearing one. I imagine a large warehouse somewhere in New York City with stacks of these shirts collecting dust.

The "I had an abortion" shirt never caught on because America is undergoing a paradigm shift in our view of abortion. Think of it like this: Men who have never owned a motorcycle will tattoo "Harley Davidson" on their arms because they want to associate with a positive symbol of Americana. But even though late-term abortionist George Tiller once hung a banner on his clinic that read "Abortion Is as American as Apple Pie," you are hard-pressed to find women who will declare publicly that they are proud of their abortions. In fact, the opposite is true. The organization Silent No More regularly holds rallies with thousands of women who are sorry they had abortions, and I have seen these women routinely displaying signs that read, "I regret my abortion."

The abortion doctors are in a similar situation. Life Dynamics Inc., a Texas pro-life group run by my good friend Mark Crutcher, conducted a survey of abortion providers several years ago. Crutcher told the *Baltimore Sun* in an article published on April 15, 1993, that results from that survey showed about 65 percent of abortion providers feel they are ostracized by their fellow physicians. Abortionists are finding it increasingly difficult to maintain hospital privileges and are being forced to "practice" abortion without the support of the medical community. They are like the bottom-feeders in a lake, lurking in the dark, scavenging for their next meal. We once knew an abortionist in San Diego who was so ashamed of his line of work that, to retain an appearance of respectability, he told his neighbors he was a weight-loss specialist.

For these reasons and more, Cheryl and I have dedicated nearly fifty years of our lives to putting these "human chop shops" out of business. We met on the streets of San Diego outside an abortion clinic (one that is now closed due to our combined efforts). Over the past two decades we have honed our skills at exposing abortionists as the "snake-oil salesmen" they truly are and in doing so have closed dozens of abortion clinics.

We are driven to shut down abortion mills because we know that when abortion clinics close, babies are spared an excruciating death, and women are protected from the predatory abortionists that exploit them when they are most vulnerable. In the early years, we would see the closure of abortion mills only in rare circumstances. However, in the last five years, we've seen more abortion mills close at a faster rate than we ever thought possible.

For decades pro-life groups have successfully lobbied for commonsense laws to protect women's health, including mandatory waiting periods and parental consent for minors seeking abortions. While we are fighting to eradicate these facilities altogether, in the meantime we feel we must do what we can to ensure the safety of the women. That is why in recent years we have successfully shifted the focus onto laws that will have an even greater impact, such as clinic licensing standards and laws requiring that abortionists maintain local hospital privileges in the event of a medical emergency. These laws have passed state legislatures because it makes sense to ensure that abortionists and facilities meet minimum safety requirements. After all, wasn't making abortion safe behind the movement to legalize abortion? Yet abortionists continue to arrogantly ignore the law even when it comes to basic practices such as clinic cleanliness, instrument sterilization, and infection control. In fact, we have yet to find an abortion business that fully complies with the law. It is probable that every abortion mill in the country should be closed due to lack of compliance with laws that are already on the books. The key is discovering and documenting what the abortionists are doing wrong, getting that information into the hands of the appropriate authorities, and then demanding enforcement. It's that simple.

There are three questions I'm often asked when discussing the concept of closing abortion clinics. The first is, "Why should we close abortion clinics?" That answer is obvious. When we close abortion clinics, we stop the infliction of human misery upon vulnerable women and their innocent babies. It's a proven fact supported by state health department abortion statistics that when abortion clinics close, fewer women have abortions.

Kansas is one state that is an example of how closing abortion clinics saves lives. Since 2001, every time an abortion clinic closed in Kansas, yearly statistics reported by the Kansas Department of Health and Environment show the number of abortions significantly dropped the following year. After the most recent clinic closure in 2009, abortions in Kansas dropped 21.3 percent over the next three years, according to KDHE statistics.

The second question I'm asked is, "Is it even possible to close these modern-day chop shops?" The answer to that is a resounding "Yes!"

For the last twenty years, we have focused the majority of our talents and time developing new strategies and tactics to close the doors of abortion mills once and for all. We have seen abortion clinics close in all fifty states and have played a direct part in closing many of them. In fact, we are writing this book from a building that was once an abortion mill where an estimated fifty thousand abortions took place. We secretly bought the building out from under the abortion business; then threw the bums out on the street. After extensive renovations, this building, once the site of so much human misery, is now our national headquarters, where our staff works tirelessly every day to stop abortion and save lives.

In the last twenty years, over 70 percent of all abortion clinics permanently closed. Since 2011, abortion clinics have been closing across the nation at the amazing rate of about two per month. This fact has put the far-left abortion crowd in a panic, and it is one of the reasons I believe Obama created the so-called Affordable Care Act, or as I call it the "Abortion Clinic Bail-Out Fund." But in spite of the best efforts of abortion apologists, lobbyists, and politicians, abortion clinics continue to close and the number of abortions continues to drop as the public becomes increasingly pro-life.

The third most common question people ask me is, "How do you close abortion clinics?" The purpose of this book is to answer this most important question. Our methods are not complicated. We have no special training beyond what we have learned through experience and from trial and error. We use strictly legal, peaceful means that anyone with a cell phone, a camera, and a computer with an Internet connection can use with very little training. Our purpose is to show you how to use these same proven methods to put abortionists out of business. We will share with you our decades of experience and explain in plain language what you can do to help close your local abortion clinic.

2

GOALS AND STRATEGIES

Setting goals is the first step in turning the invisible into the visible.

—**TONY ROBBINS**

If you are reading this book, then you likely are a champion of life and want to do something to end the culture of death that pervades our country. When you make the decision to get involved, you have to prepare yourself. As Julie Andrew sang in *The Sound of Music,* "Let's start at the very beginning, a very good place to start." Before taking any action, you must create a mind-set where success is inevitable. You have to believe that it is possible and commit yourself to the goal of stopping abortion in your community. That sounds obvious, but as my dad is fond of saying, "Sometimes the obvious needs to be stated."

Without a goal, it is impossible to focus efforts or measure your success. Approach the project with the resolve that you will never stop employing every peaceful, legal, and moral tool at your disposal until the local abortion mill has permanently closed and decide from the get-go that failure is not an option.

It is important to set modest, intermediate goals that will put you in position for decisive victory. If there is more than one abortion clinic in your community, you may want do a bit of preliminary research to determine the weakest one or the one with the most problems and focus there first. We call this picking the low-lying fruit. This is a way to quickly reduce abortions in your community, and in doing so, give encouragement to your fellow activists that the task of making your community abortion-free is a doable one.

Once you have begun, it's important to periodically measure your success. Make note of what has worked and what hasn't. Tracking your goals and acknowledging your short-term victories will encourage you and set you up for further success.

Back in the early 1990s, a team of five of us held a planning meeting in Cheryl's home. We set a goal to stop the abortion industry in San Diego. After five years of working the plan, we were able to look back and see that eighteen abortion mills had shut down. That triumph helped propel us to even more victories and let us know we were on the right track.

As you work toward your goals, you, too, will begin to see mile markers of success. Maybe there will be a decrease in the number of abortion patients or the number of days when abortions are offered by the clinic. You may notice that the clinic struggles to keep vendors or suffers financial setbacks. You may see a high staff turnover, or clinic workers walking off the job to join you on the sidewalk. But no matter how small the victories, never lose sight of the ultimate goal. Once you are armed with a goal, you can begin to map out a strategy to accomplish it.

Strategy is the means with which to accomplish a goal, and *tactics* are the detailed way to employ the means. Think of strategy as a toolbox and tactics as the individual tools. If you have a leaky water heater, your goal is to repair the leak. The *strategy* would be to use your tools to accomplish the goal, and your *tactics* are the correct use of each tool to accomplish the repair.

When we set out to close Phillip Milgram's two abortion mills in San Diego County, our strategy was to apply pressure outside his clinic every day he was open. Our tactics involved confronting every potential customer and abortion-bound mom with a flyer that documented his misdeeds and showed a graphic picture of an aborted baby.

The use of strategies is both an art and a science. About two abortion clinics per month are closing right now in the United States, but each is closing for different reasons. Every city and every state are different, and all have a variety of laws, so a strategy that works very well in Nebraska may not work at all in New York City. In some states you may be successful with a legislative strategy that will not work in states that require a more activist approach. In the same way, tactics that work on one clinic may not work on another, even in the same city. In that case, the strategy may not change, but it may be essential to adjust your tactics. We must use the right tools from the right toolbox to get the job done successfully.

In Kansas, we scored a hat trick when we closed three separate abortion clinics within a five-year time frame. Each clinic had its own unique issues. While we employed the same persistent strategy, we used very different tactics to close each clinic.

Kristin Neuhaus was forced to close her abortion mill in Lawrence, Kansas, after the Board of Healing Arts received complaints. The board forced a temporary closure after they found the clinic was guilty of dangerously inadequate record keeping. Neuhaus reopened after six weeks but had lost too much business to remain open. She told the *Lawrence Journal-World*, "We had no income for six weeks, which is over 10 percent of the year, and then the weeks following that we had 25 percent loss for the rest of the year" ("Lawrence abortion clinic closes because of funding woes," September 11, 2002, http://www2.ljworld.com/news/2002/sep/11/lawrence_abortion_clinic_closes/).

Due to complaints driven by pro-life supporters, she was forced to close her doors for good.

The second victory in our hat trick was the closing of Affordable Medical Clinic, operated by Krishna Rajanna of Kansas City. Pro-life sidewalk counselors had persuaded a disgruntled employee to photograph the horrific conditions inside the clinic. They provided the worker with a disposable camera on her way into the clinic for her shift. Secretly, she photographed the appalling conditions. As she left for the day, she returned the camera to an awaiting sidewalk counselor. The photos were turned over to authorities and presented to the legislature in support of proposed clinic regulations. Kansas City detective William Howard, who witnessed what can only be described as a "house of horrors" during an investigation he conducted at the clinic, submitted written testimony concerning the horrible conditions to the Kansas House Committee on Health and Human Services, which was considering a bill to license clinics and set minimum safety standards.

Howard noted that "the doctor was unkempt, with dirty hands, messy hair, and stained clothing." Howard described the clinic as "dark and dingy" and that it smelled "musty." He reported that there were dirty dishes in the sink, trash was everywhere, roaches were crawling across the counters, and there were no visible medical waste containers. Employees from the clinic reported that Rajanna would take all the medical waste home. Howard's partner also reported seeing dried blood on the carpeted floor of a "nasty"-looking procedure room.

Howard stated that he learned from interviews with clinic employees that abortion equipment was sterilized by washing it in a dishwasher with Clorox. It was also reported that aborted fetuses were placed in Styrofoam cups next to TV dinners in the refrigerator. Howard also testified that several female witnesses reported having seen Rajanna "microwave a fetus and stir it into his lunch" (March 15, 2005, http://operationrescue.org/files/dethoward.pdf).

You might not think that abortion clinics can get that bad in this day of modern medical advances, but our research has shown that the conditions found at Rajanna's abortion mill are hardly anomalous, as was tragically proven in 2011 when police raided Kermit Gosnell's abortion clinic. The prosecutor expected to find a pill mill, but instead he was confronted with Rajanna-like conditions and the discovery of unspeakable abortion horrors that led to Gosnell's conviction on three counts of first-degree murder, involuntary manslaughter, infanticide, and literally hundreds of other violations of the Abortion Control Act of Pennsylvania.

Once the truth about Rajanna's squalid clinic and appalling practices reached the public, the Kansas Board of Healing Arts finally acted to revoke his medical license and closed the mill for good, all because pro-life supporters worked a strategy that achieved their goal.

The final success in our Kansas hat trick was putting Wichita's Central Women's Services out of business. We applied consistent on-site pressure, and then watched for a moment of opportunity. In a surprisingly short amount of time, we noticed that the clinic was rapidly going downhill. We carefully monitored activity at the clinic and discovered it had a high turnover of abortion workers and providers. The clinic was staffed by abortionists from the Kansas City area three hours away. These abortionists obviously hated the long drive to Wichita. We knew from our observations about how many abortions were being done per month, and after doing some quick math, we realized that the abortionists came to town less frequently than was needed for financial solvency. It was easy to see the clinic was losing money.

Then came the moment of opportunity. Through an anonymous tip we learned that the building owner had grown impatient with late or nonexistent rent payments from the abortion business and had placed the building up for sale, thinking he would sell only to a "pro-choice" buyer. We immediately made an offer through a third party and closed the deal.

Once the abortion business found out the building had sold, they asked to retain tenancy. Of course, we refused and forced them to vacate the building before the end of escrow. The clinic was broke and without capital reserves; moving was not an option. The business folded.

One hat trick in the bag.

We are excited to share our strategies and the tactics that have been so successful. We hope you will use our experiences as a reference to guide and inspire you as you work to stop abortion in your community.

In the following pages we will discuss how to do undercover investigations to find the hidden secrets the abortion industry wants no one to know. We will show you how to make formal complaints to medical boards and how to interface directly with investigators and prosecutors. You will learn how to persuade authorities to enforce the law against abortion clinics and providers that routinely act as though they are above the law.

We have assisted legislatures in passing abortion laws that have "teeth," and we want to enable you to be able to look a lawmaker in the eye and confidently explain how the abortion cartel is getting away with murder, and exactly what he or she must do about it.

If simple people like us can close countless abortion clinics, I assure you that with a little help, you can make your city abortion-free. In all our combined decades of experience, we have yet to find an abortion business that abides by all applicable laws. That means every abortion clinic is legally vulnerable and subject to closure. Our job is to find out what the abortionists are doing wrong and exploit their weaknesses.

In 1991, there were 2,176 abortion clinics in the United States. We know this because Life Dynamics Inc. had conducted a survey of abortion clinics that year. We then had a gauge with which we could measure the pro-life movement's level of success.

In 2010, we began conducting our own survey of abortion clinics and have kept it current. In December 2013, our office conducted an exhaustive survey of existing abortion clinics in the United States. We expected to double the twenty-four abortion clinics known to have closed in 2012, but what we actually found stunned us. In 2013, an astounding eighty-seven surgical abortion clinics closed their doors for good. (Eleven others were shut down for a portion of the year, but managed to find a way to reopen.) In addition, six clinics that offered abortions only via the RU-486 abortion pill also permanently closed, making a grand total of ninety-three abortion facilities out of business in one year alone. As of January 2014, the number of surgical abortion clinics had plummeted to 581. This is a decline of 73 percent since 1991. As you can see, the pro-life movement—often without realizing it—is nearing its goal of closing every abortion clinic in the country. Less than 30 percent of the work remains.

Our experiences and successes confirm that our tactics work, and at no place was this more apparent than in Wichita, Kansas, where we put them to the ultimate test.

PART 2

A CASE STUDY: WICHITA, KANSAS

3

"COME TO WICHITA"

Rescue those being led away to death; hold back those staggering toward slaughter. If you say, "But we knew nothing about this," does not he who weighs the heart perceive it? Does not he who guards your life know it? Will he not repay everyone according to what they have done?

—**PROVERBS 24:11–12**

After living in Southern California all my life, I sold my property, loaded my family into a motor home, and headed for Kansas. It was 2002.

I was convinced that we should use the tactics we had developed in Southern California to focus on the most notorious abortion clinic in the nation. If we could close that clinic down, it would give hope to everyone in the pro-life movement.

That clinic was George Tiller's Women's Health Care Services (WHCS) in Wichita.

I was raised in San Diego and enjoyed a "surfer boy" lifestyle in my youth. Even after marriage, my wife, Mellissa, and I were attracted to the lifestyle of the upscale beach communities. Yet, so strong was God's call on my life that I was willing to leave the familiar comforts of California and relocate my growing family to Kansas.

After our experiences in Southern California and the success we enjoyed there, I thought we could accomplish our goal of closing the country's most infamous abortion clinic in a year or two. Because we'd closed so many California clinics and encouraged multiple abortionists to leave the killing business, I had every reason for optimism as I drove east on I-40, then north at Tucumcari, New Mexico, onto Highway 54, which would take us eventually right past Tiller's Wichita clinic.

But I was not prepared for the reception I received upon my arrival. I believed Operation Rescue would be welcomed with open arms by the local pro-lifers, but instead, to my surprise, I was met with jealousy and suspicion from those who were not open to change or new ideas. Many believed that since the clinic had been there "forever," it was doubtful that our tactics could work. When I told them we could indeed close Tiller's abortion clinic, they scoffed. They rejected the plan and they rejected me.

Given the previous history in Wichita, it was easy to see why they felt that way.

In 1991, Operation Rescue's Summer of Mercy protests landed Wichita at the epicenter of the abortion wars, making national headlines with more than twenty-six hundred arrests for peaceful civil disobedience. For six weeks, thousands of pro-lifers from across America, from nearly every walk of life, descended on Wichita to participate in the "rescue missions" that primarily focused on Tiller's late-term abortion clinic. Men and women—even children—peacefully blocked the entrance to Tiller's clinic and those of two other abortion clinics operating in Wichita at that time.

Federal court judge Patrick Kelly tried to put an end to the protests with his famous message to pro-life supporters during a national television news interview that was widely quoted in newspaper articles around the country. Though the transcript does not seem to be available online, I have a scanned news clipping from the *Nevada Daily*

Mail, dated August 6, 1991, in which the judge told the Associated Press, "They [pro-life demonstrators] should say farewell to their family and bring a toothbrush, and I mean it, because they are going to jail. It's that simple."

Instead of deterring those of conviction, Kelly's threats emboldened the pro-life movement. Pastors preached from the pulpits about abortion, some for the first time. Dr. James Dobson dedicated several of his popular Focus on the Family radio shows to coverage of the Summer of Mercy and encouraged Christians to essentially drop everything and go to Wichita to save babies from abortion.

The protests blocked streets, bogged down the court system, and created uproar in the community. The personal sacrifices of these Christians were successful at closing Tiller's clinic for a glorious eleven days and saved more than ninety babies from abortion.

But after six weeks, the protesters left town. Tiller reopened his clinic and continued business as usual.

The Summer of Mercy taught Tiller an important lesson. All he had to do was outlast the latest pro-life event, after which he could resume his abortion business without much opposition. That was a lesson that, unfortunately, we reinforced for him again and again.

He could afford patience. His late-term procedures, which cost between five thousand and eighteen thousand dollars—or more—had made him a rich man. Money is power, and Tiller knew that better than most. He used his wealth to accrue political favors, which ensured that he was able to operate with very little oversight or accountability. He hired a phalanx of attorneys to tend to his legal issues and intimidate his opposition inside the government. He successfully presented himself as the victim of lawless antiabortionists and gained sympathy in the community.

In 1994, Tiller dramatically expanded his office building, making it the largest free-standing late-term abortion clinic outside of

Communist China. The local pro-life activists could do little to prevent it. They soon settled into a peaceful coexistence with the most notorious abortion clinic in the world!

On the tenth anniversary of the Summer of Mercy, Operation Rescue once again led protests at Tiller's abortion clinic. This time, the event was attended by hundreds instead of thousands, lasted only one week, and resulted in two arrests that were staged for the news media. Tiller patiently outlasted the event as he had the others. It did little to impact Tiller's immediate business. For all intents and purposes, Tiller and his staff thought it was over when Operation Rescue left town in July 2001.

Little did they know it was just the beginning.

Cheryl and I were present at the 2001 event. I was the newly installed leader of Operation Rescue West, based in the sunbaked mountains of Southern California near Lake Arrowhead. We believed that if we could keep consistent, California-style pressure on Tiller's clinic, the abortion clinic would soon close. To keep up that pressure, we knew we had to move to Kansas. That's why in 2002 I packed up my growing young family and headed east. Cheryl's oldest daughter, Brenna, who was my administrative assistant, also moved to Wichita with my family.

Cheryl resisted the call to Kansas at first. She had founded and was leading a thriving pro-life ministry in San Diego, called the California Life Coalition. Her efforts at sidewalk counseling had spared more than twenty-five hundred babies from abortion. She was open to using new ideas and tactics in combination with tried-and-true methods to impact the abortion cartel, and together we had witnessed the closure of multiple abortion clinics in our area.

I knew about Cheryl's past but understood it was just that—the past. In 1987, she and several members of her church at that time had been involved in a conspiracy to damage an abortion clinic in San Diego. There was never any damage done. Among those involved in the scheme was her pastor, Dorman Owens. A friend and fellow church member, Eric Svelmoe, was caught in the act, and Cheryl, her husband, and five others were arrested and charged with helping him. She took full responsibility for her part in the debacle and spent two years in a federal prison in Lexington, Kentucky, far from her home and family in San Diego.

Since then, Cheryl has dedicated herself to peaceful, legal activism to close abortion clinics, something that has been much more successful than any attempt to use violence ever was. Ironically, while she has helped to close dozens of abortion clinics through her legal efforts, the clinic that was the subject of the conspiracy remains open to this day.

Certainly the abortion crowd never lets her forget this admitted mistake she made decades ago. However, I have always believed that if we in the pro-life movement can forgive and embrace women who have had abortions, as well as those, like former Planned Parenthood director Abby Johnson and Dr. Anthony Levatino, who actually participated in the killing of innocent children by abortion, then we should also be able to forgive those in our own ranks who have made mistakes but have repented and amended their ways.

In 1993, a list of more than seventy abortionists working in San Diego County was published in a monthly Catholic newspaper called the *San Diego News Notes*. I remember sitting in a pro-life strategy meeting at Cheryl's house, thinking that the list was a gift from God to help us expose the abortionists and close their clinics. As a first step, we sent letters to each abortionist, asking the physician to quit the abortion business and use his or her talents instead for healing—or be subject to a public information campaign.

We would never recommend such a foolish ultimatum today. It embroiled us in a lawsuit with a Planned Parenthood abortionist that resulted in ten years of legal battles. That decade of litigation could have been avoided if we had used language that did not include the threat of exposure through picketing if the clinics did not stop their abortion practice. It would have been better to just politely ask them to stop doing abortions and let them know we were praying for them. It was a costly lesson for us that diverted precious time away from our work to stop abortion, not to mention the personal financial drain that none of us could really afford.

Nevertheless, several abortionists quit on the spot. Several others left the abortion industry after we assembled our people and conducted regular prayer pickets in their neighborhoods. Many of these clinicians did not want their neighbors to know what they did for a living. One told his neighbors that he was a weight-loss specialist. Another said he was a brain surgeon. Abortionists understand that their line of work carries a stigma. When we told the truth about them, many decided that performing abortions wasn't worth the tarnishing of their reputations.

In 1999 Operation Rescue celebrated ten years of ministry in Southern California. Looking back on our accomplishments, we were shocked to discover that, out of the seventy abortionists we wrote to in 1993, only about forty remained. We had been so busy focusing on the work we had left to do that we did not realize how much we had accomplished.

We now had quantifiable evidence that our tactics and methods worked.

I wanted to take the knowledge and experience we had acquired on the streets of Southern California and apply it in Kansas. I had envisioned the Wichita project as being a model on which others could pattern their efforts to close abortion clinics around the country.

After hearing of the resistance I faced in Wichita and knowing she could help the work get done, Cheryl broached the idea of moving to Kansas with her husband, Randy. To her surprise, he agreed it was a great idea. That was in June 2003. By September, the Sullenger family had pulled in the driveway of their new Wichita home after having sold their East San Diego County condo for top dollar just months before the real estate bubble burst in Southern California. We could see plainly that the hand of God was at work bringing all the elements together for success.

Establishing the work in Wichita was no easy task. We had to overcome small-minded, parochial thinking of activists who simply did not want to make changes. Worse, many of the local pro-life "leaders" began to actively undermine our work. It showed me the ugly side of pro-life turf wars, which was a painful and difficult thing for me to cope with on a personal basis.

As in Nehemiah's time, the Sanballat, Tobiah, and Geshem types were feigning spirituality while sowing division and discord in an effort to undermine our work. I learned a lot from the biblical book of Nehemiah during that time. Those naysayers wanted me to give up, but instead, we made every effort to ignore them and focus instead on our goal.

Don't think when you start a new work in your community that there won't be opposition! Unfortunately, some individuals and/or groups will see you as competition that must be crushed. So it was with us in Wichita.

In the end, we were forced to separate from those who were undermining our work. We ignored the naysayers as best we could and labored on with a coalition of the willing that grew as time went by.

4

FIRST THINGS FIRST

It is said that if you know your enemies and know yourself, you will not be imperiled in a hundred battles; if you do not know your enemies but do know yourself, you will win one and lose one; if you do not know your enemies nor yourself, you will be imperiled in every single battle.

—**SUN TZU, *THE ART OF WAR***

The first thing we did in Wichita was opposition research. We needed to know as much as we could about Tiller's abortion business. Why did he choose to become an abortionist? What were his affiliations? How did his abortion clinic operate? Who worked for him, and who were his vendors?

To find the answers, we had to wade through the folklore and rumors that permeated the local pro-life movement and try to find the hard, documentable facts. We had a rule that has remained with us to this day: if there is no document to back up an allegation, we won't put it in print.

It took us about a year not only to research Tiller but to learn how things worked in Kansas. Every state has its own unique set of abortion laws and regulatory system. We expended time and effort to understand who was responsible for which aspect of abortion oversight and who the major influencers were when it came to the matter of abortion.

Once we were sure of our facts, we developed a plan.

First, we published *The Tiller Report,* a seventy-two-page booklet that detailed Tiller's history as an abortionist, the inner workings of his business, and his place in the community. We identified his clinic workers, charities he supported with donations, and where his campaign contributions went.

Unlike most abortionists, who tend to live on the fringes of society, Tiller was remarkably well connected and respected in his community. He was a wealthy man who used his wealth to buy the esteem of others. He served as an usher in his church. He gave money to charity. He operated a very effective political action committee that helped shift his very red home state to blue in 2002, with the election of the radically pro-abortion Democrat Kathleen Sebelius as governor.

We were determined to use what we had learned about him and his shocking late-term abortion business and practices to turn public opinion against him. We committed our plan to prayer, then braced for the ride of our lives. It was time to launch our first major offensive.

In January 2004 we held a press conference and announced a controversial new project. We called it "the Year of Rebuke." We revealed our plan to expose the dirt on Tiller and his late-term baby-killing operation as no one had ever done before. We displayed a graphic that we labeled "Tiller's Web of Death," which showed the layers of support Tiller had developed, starting with his inner circle of clinic workers and encompassing the hospital where he held privileges, as well as other business and political cronies.

We admit the language was a bit strident, but it certainly got everyone's attention. Shortly afterwards, I was contacted by the *Los Angeles Times,* who wanted to do a feature article on me and the Year of Rebuke campaign. *Times* reporter Stephanie Simon came to Kansas for several days, spending time with us at our office and accompanying us during our pro-life outreaches. She also interviewed Tiller's clinic administrator, Carrie Klaege, who had been the subject of Operation Rescue's Year of Rebuke prayer vigils.

We regularly parked the Truth Truck, bearing large, graphic images of aborted babies, at the entrance to Klaege's upscale Bel Aire neighborhood on the northeastern outskirts of Wichita. Everyone who lived beyond the "choke point" had to pass by the Truth Truck every morning on the way to work and each evening on the way home. It created quite a stir in that quiet neighborhood.

One cold winter evening, we conducted one of our prayer walks in Klaege's neighborhood. It was our policy to always leave together and never allow stragglers to stay behind. There was safety in numbers, and lone pro-lifers in hostile territory were at risk of false accusations or even physical attacks that would never occur to a larger group. That evening, something happened that reinforced the necessity of our "no man left behind" policy.

As we jumped into our cars and left the area, I noticed the flashing lights of a police cruiser closing in on our Truth Truck. I pulled over to make sure everything was okay with our truck and driver. Concerned, Cheryl pulled in behind me with her camera at the ready to document the incident.

The Bel Aire police had stopped the Truth Truck just outside Klaege's neighborhood and began to give our driver grief over the truck's California tags. Even though the tags were current, the police accused him of driving without a valid registration. After some debate, the chief of police ordered one of his officers to remove the license plate from the back of the Truth Truck. Cheryl snapped photos of the officer literally stealing our license plate while the chief unsuccessfully attempted to block her camera angle! Our driver received a ticket for driving the truck without a valid vehicle tag. Banned from driving the Truth Truck any farther, we were forced to call a tow truck and have it hauled out of Bel Aire.

To expose this injustice, we posted a photo on Operation Rescue's website of the officer in the act of removing our license plate. The police department's phone lines lit up with calls complaining about their shameful behavior.

Tensions in the community grew, and it became clear that city officials would go to any lengths to keep us out of Bel Aire. Our Truth Truck was repeatedly vandalized. Once the windows were smashed; another time our signs were covered with spray paint. Our tires were slashed. We simply made the repairs, ordered new signs, and got the Truth Truck back out on the street as soon as possible.

Finally, everything came to a head when I was falsely arrested and charged for violating the fashionable community's building code restricting the use of portable signs. We publicly denounced the trumped-up charges and the continuing persecution from the Bel Aire police.

Anticipating that I was about to get the "book" thrown at me, local reporters and camera crews packed the tiny court building for my hearing. Apparently, city officials finally realized that the city faced a potential First Amendment lawsuit that could draw unwanted national attention to their brazenly illegal acts. My case was immediately dismissed without so much as a comment—much less an apology.

Klaege told the *Times* reporter of our neighborhood presence, "If their point is to get us to quit, this is probably the worst way to go about it" (Stephanie Simon, "Protestors Who Push the Limits," *Los Angeles Times*, February 17, 2004, http://articles.latimes.com/2004/feb/17/nation/na-abortion17).

But within weeks, Klaege had traded her job at Tiller's clinic for work at a candle shop in the mall. Her absence left a personnel void that Tiller struggled to fill.

The *Los Angeles Times* article was a boon for us. It painted a picture of determined activists who were not about to give up and go away. That story led to a call from *Rolling Stone* magazine, which ran a feature article on me called "One Man's God Squad" that spotlighted our work in Wichita (Kimberley Sevcik, 2004). After the *Rolling Stone* article was published, the Tiller story caught the eye of Fox News personality Bill O'Reilly. Tiller's horrific late-term abortion business became national news once again.

5

GAME CHANGER

Be prepared in season and out of season . . . —**2 TIMOTHY 4:2**

Just days before our 2005 *Roe v. Wade* events were to begin, an unexpected event gave our project a greater sense of urgency and relevance.

Our phones began to ring shortly after 8:00 a.m. on the frigid but sunny morning of January 13, 2005. Sidewalk counselors at Tiller's clinic reported that an ambulance had arrived. That alone was not such an uncommon occurrence. We had documented several such incidents over the preceding months.

We had a system in place for responding to calls like this. We kept our cameras charged and at the ready. Cheryl kept a tripod in the trunk of her car. When the calls came in, some staffers rushed to Tiller's clinic, while others made a mad dash for Wesley Medical Center, where Tiller transported all his botched abortion patients.

Our response system was a well-oiled machine that came about from far too much practice. Ambulances at Tiller's late-term abortion clinic were an all-too-common sight. When we first came to Wichita, local activists told us that ambulances came to the clinic all the time, but there was nothing we could do about it.

We had been shocked by that attitude of resignation to the life-threatening injuries of so many women. There certainly *was* something that could be done about it!

We dropped everything to rush to the scene and document these incidents. Some of us would dash off to the clinic, if we weren't there already. Others of our staff made a beeline for the hospital. We videotaped and snapped photos as fast as we could.

In June 2004, we had been milling about the clinic, waiting for abortion-bound women to arrive so we could offer them help, when an ambulance pulled into the parking lot. With the excitement of the moment taking over, I ran to the ditch behind Tiller's clinic and began snapping photos of the back entrance over the six-foot-tall fence, hoping I didn't slip and fall into the murky water that flowed through the flood control channel just a few feet below me. Cheryl ran to the porch of Choices Medical Center, a pro-life clinic directly next door to Tiller's clinic, where she shot video from one of the best vantage points available to us. As the ambulance pulled out with the poor, injured woman who'd come to Tiller for an abortion, we dashed to our cars in hot pursuit.

We arrived at Wesley Medical Center, where Tiller sent all his botched abortion patients for emergency medical care, and began to snap photos while the emergency medical technicians rushed the gurney into the emergency room.

Afterwards, anxious to see how our pictures turned out, we hurried our cameras to Cheryl's house, where she had a fully functional office. We quickly downloaded the pictures from the digital camera and opened the files. All of a sudden we both screamed in surprise!

What we thought was one of the EMTs was actually George Tiller himself. We had caught amazing pictures of him jumping out of the ambulance and pushing his wounded patient into the hospital.

It was the best-documented medical emergency at an abortion clinic that we had ever seen. There was no denying that this was a Tiller patient who required emergency hospitalization. It was hard proof that something dangerous was happening at that infamous late-term abortion clinic that pro-abortion politicians had said was the best in the world.

We took the best of those pictures, enlarged it, mounted it on the side of the Truth Truck, and drove it all over town. We also parked it outside the clinic gate, where abortion-bound women couldn't miss it. Many babies were saved from abortion after women saw that image and decided not to take the risk of ending up like the girl on the gurney.

Over the next few years, we documented about a dozen and a half such medical emergencies and used that evidence to call for abortion safety reforms. Eventually, Tiller changed his emergency protocols and stopped calling for ambulances, opting instead to dangerously smuggle injured women past the pro-life presence outside his clinic and to the hospital in private vehicles.

So it was that on January 13, 2005, Cheryl and Brenna responded to what had become the routine call from the sidewalk counselors reporting an ambulance on-site at Tiller's abortion clinic.

The ladies arrived at Wesley that cold January morning just as paramedics were off-loading the gurney carrying the injured abortion patient. The grim-faced emergency workers, seemingly on the edge of panic, hastily slid the gurney from the tailgate and rushed the patient to the hospital emergency room entrance. Brenna sensed the heightened tensions as she snapped still photos with trembling hands.

Cheryl and Brenna knew there was something different about this incident. They worried that the unknown patient had suffered more serious abortion complications than usual. They wondered if she had died. Later, we dropped our usual post-abortion-injury press release decrying the dangers of Tiller's late-term abortion procedure, which, as usual, was ignored by the local media.

But those concerns were put temporarily on hold as we busied ourselves with a full slate of events that were planned for *Roe v. Wade* week that year. After our Monday press conference, we planned a Tuesday morning protest outside the La Quinta Inn where Tiller stabled his late-term patients and overnight staff. On Wednesday, six days after the ambulance incident, we were scheduled to protest Wesley Medical Center for their collaboration in Tiller's abortion practice.

While picketing outside Wesley, a Wichita Police officer approached me and asked to speak with me privately. Wondering what trouble I was in this time, I followed the officer over to an empty parking lot near an abandoned business down the street. The officer had seen our press releases concerning the most recent abortion emergency at Tiller's clinic and wanted to let me know that the woman transported to Wesley on the thirteenth had died.

Even with the word of a police officer, whose identity we have protected all these years, we were still uncomfortable about releasing the news to the press because we had no hard documentation.

Two days later, we visited the office of the governor and spoke with Vicki Buening, who served as Governor Sebelius's director of constituent services. When showed a number of photos of several ambulance runs from Tiller's Women's Health Care Services to the local hospital, Mrs. Buening told me that if women were unhappy with the care they received at WHCS, they were free to file a complaint with the Kansas State Board of Healing Arts.

What we didn't know at that time was that Mrs. Buening was the wife of Larry Buening, who was then the executive director of the Kansas State Board of Healing Arts. Mr. Buening had worked closely with Tiller years before, helping him preserve his medical career when Tiller was battling substance abuse. The two were fast friends.

The following is a partial transcript of an exchange we videotaped and archived between a visibly nervous Vicki Buening and Cheryl during that meeting:

> **Buening:** Now individuals involved in any of these kinds of mishandling of their medical care have the option to file a complaint against their provider with the Board of Healing Arts.
>
> **Sullenger:** If they're still alive.
>
> **Buening:** Certainly that is true. Whether, uh—[pause]. Yeah, you're right. But I, uh . . .
>
> **Sullenger:** If they are dead, they can't file a complaint, can they?
>
> **Buening:** I don't have an answer to that question.

Our mention of a hypothetical abortion death prompted an unexpected reaction. We sensed that Buening was aware of the abortion death but was attempting to hide it.

Four days after the meeting with Buening, we decided to go public with what we knew. We dropped a press release announcing that Operation Rescue had been informed that an abortion patient from Women's Health Care Services had died. We publicly called on the Kansas State Board of Healing Arts (KSBHA) to investigate.

Within minutes of pushing the send button, Cheryl's cell phone rang. It was Shelly Wakeman, disciplinary attorney with the KSBHA. She explained that without a formal complaint, there was nothing the board could do. Wakeman directed Cheryl to the official KSBHA online complaint form. She printed it out, filled it in, and faxed it to the KSBHA. Minutes later, Wakeman faxed a letter back to her acknowledging her complaint and confirming that Tiller was now under investigation.

We learned then to never underestimate the power of a formal complaint filed on a regulatory agency's official complaint form. Once such a complaint is logged into the system, it initiates a process that takes on a life of its own. It is a serious matter, and Tiller would have a lot of explaining to do. Because of that, it caught the attention of Governor Sebelius, who immediately went into damage-control mode.

Sebelius again sent a letter to Larry Buening, the KSBHA's executive director, asking him to look into the death at WHCS, even though she was well aware of the Operation Rescue complaint. In addition to protecting the abortionists responsible for the patient death, she was battling a clinic licensing and regulations bill that had been introduced in the legislature following our revelations of so many life-threatening patient injuries that were taking place at the Wichita abortion clinic.

Something had to be done to prevent the patient tragedy in Wichita from becoming the rallying cry for abortion clinic accountability. We later found out the hard way how much influence Sebelius had acquired within oversight agencies in Kansas, and how committed she was to ensuring that late-term abortions continued unimpeded by regulation or law—whatever the cost.

We knew we needed to get the victim's autopsy report, not only to discover the truth about what happened to the dead patient, but also to buttress our accusations that Tiller's clinic was engaged in a shoddy and possibly illegal abortion enterprise that posed a danger to the public. We called the medical examiner's office to request a copy but were told that without the patient's name, nothing could be released.

How in the world were we going to find that out? The Bible teaches in James 4:2 that when we do not have, it is because we did not ask, so we decided to start asking.

We made a flurry of open records requests to various city agencies for information, but nothing turned up. Determined to find out the victim's name, Cheryl went to the Sedgwick County Courthouse and began a tedious and systematic search of each document filed with the court in numerical sequence beginning on January 1, 2005. After hours of blurry-eyed scanning of everything from criminal cases to divorce filings, finally a document popped up that sent her heart racing.

It was a subpoena for medical records from Wesley Medical Center, issued by a judge in Tarrant County, Texas, on behalf of a grand jury investigating the sexual assault of a nineteen-year-old girl with Down syndrome who died of injuries related to a third-trimester abortion at Wesley on January 13, 2005.

We finally had a name: Christin Alysabeth Gilbert.

Cheryl held her breath and pressed the print button. Clutching the document, she hurried out of the courthouse as quickly as she dared, fearing that someone would realize what she had discovered and seize the paper before she could reach the safety of her "getaway" car. Media reports had earlier indicated that Tiller's records had been subpoenaed by the Texas grand jury, but there was no trace of Tiller's subpoena in the system.

We believe to this day that there was an attempt by someone in the county government to expunge the record of the subpoenas in order to protect Tiller. The Wesley document had simply been overlooked. That was no accident; it was divine providence!

Our research discovered that Christin Alysabeth Gilbert was born on May 30, 1985, in Austin, Texas, but spent most of her life in the small Texas town of Keller. Even though Christin had Down syndrome, it did not stop her from embracing life and living it to the fullest. Christin enjoyed family life with her mom, dad, and older sister.

Christin became involved in sports early in her life because it helped her meet people and make friends. She became very active in the Special Olympics and participated proudly for ten years. In 2003 she won the gold medal in the softball throw.

Christin graduated from the special education program of Keller High School in 2004. While in high school, Christin joined the girls' softball team as the batgirl and became the inspiration to her classmates. Team members were never "allowed" to become discouraged during a tough game because Christin would meet them at the dugout with hugs, telling them that she loved them. This kept spirits high, and eventually her team won a state championship, an accomplishment of which Christin and her family were especially proud.

In life, Christin was a joy to be around. Everyone who came near her became the recipient of her many hugs. She was the center of attention when she walked into a room because of her happy-go-lucky, outgoing, and loving spirit.

Christin was loved by all who knew her, and her death left a void in the lives of her family and community. She was cremated, and a private funeral service was held for her in her hometown of Keller, Texas, on January 21, 2005. In her obituary, Christin was called "one of God's angels." The 2005 Keller Special Olympics was dedicated to her memory.

Christin was a true victim of abortion. She never made a "choice" in any abortion-related thing that happened to her. She was impregnated during a sexual assault; then she was forced to endure an abortion that painfully took her life. Often we hear from coldhearted pro-lifers such appalling statements as "Women who have abortions deserve to burn in hell." (Don't we all deserve that fate because of our sinful natures?) Certainly we all must bear responsibility and consequences for our actions, but this harsh, unforgiving attitude toward women who have abortions betrays a lack of compassion and understanding of the complex and often coercive circumstances with which pregnant women must cope.

In Christin Gilbert's case, we had none of those concerns. She was an innocent victim in every way, and maybe that is why so many people rallied around efforts to seek justice for her. Even Christin's paternal grandmother was supportive of our efforts and supplied us with precious family photos that chronicled Christin's all-too-short life.

There is no doubt that Cheryl's research efforts, which finally yielded Gilbert's name, were mind-numbingly tedious and time-consuming, but this is the kind of work that is often necessary in order to achieve results. Sometimes the things we have to do to get the job done are not exciting or glamorous. Most people would have given up or not bothered in the first place, but it is often the grueling "grunt work" that proves to be the most critical part of pro-life work.

6

911—NO LIGHTS, NO SIRENS

"Sir, I'm sorry but I don't have that information."

—**TILLER EMPLOYEE MARGUERITE REED TO EMERGENCY DISPATCHER, JANUARY 13, 2005**

Next in importance to obtaining Christin Gilbert's name was the acquisition of the 911 audio record and the computer-aided dispatch, or CAD, transcript. The CAD document is a written record of the emergency dispatcher's interaction with the caller and responding assets, such as fire and ambulance units. CADs create a timeline of events and give a different perspective to the incident than that provided by the recorded call.

Open records requests were made for the 911 records, and the Office of Emergency Communications happily complied. However, once we released the recording to the public, that was the last recording we ever got from them.

Sebelius's political network worked overtime to protect Tiller. One of her main allies in Wichita was district attorney Nola Foulston, truly the queen of her realm. Foulston "ruled the roost" at the

Sedgwick County Courthouse with dictatorial power. There is no doubt that Foulston's pro-Tiller policies were behind the illegal blocking of our later 911 requests.

Why would she intervene in such a mundane matter as a public document request? It was long rumored that Foulston's son, now an adult, was adopted from Tiller, who used to arrange such adoptions to curry political favors and loyalty. He boasted of as much in a newspaper interview that appeared in the *Oklahoman* in December 1993.

"Anti-abortion folks never get an opportunity to adopt," Tiller stated regarding his adoption practices. "I've got to know you or you've got to be important to some of my friends who have supported our family and our goals for a long period of time . . . It helps me pay back in kind the people who have supported our program."

His "program" was the business of late-term abortions, from which Christin Gilbert would later die.

But when the Gilbert 911 records were released, the Tiller cover-up machine was not yet cranking at the Sedgwick County Department of Emergency Communications.

I anxiously popped the disk into the computer and clicked the play button. What I heard on the recording was stunning.

Tiller employee Marguerite Reed, a thirtysomething married gal who worked for Tiller primarily as a receptionist, placed the call at 8:48 a.m. on that frosty January morning in 2005. Her voice was pleading, but not with any sense of urgency over the condition of the poor girl who lay dying. Her primary concern was that the ambulance might alert pro-life activists that a serious emergency was in progress.

"But please, please, please! No lights and no sirens!" she pleaded on the recording to the 911 dispatcher.

"Ma'am, I can't control that," the dispatcher responded. "And what's the problem? Tell me exactly what happened."

"This is the correct number for the ambulance, right?" Reed asked.

Correct number for the ambulance? Was she kidding? She had just dialed 911. The conversation seemed unbelievable.

"Yes, ma'am. What's the problem? Tell me exactly what happened," the dispatcher repeated.

"Okay, all I know is that it's a patient who has to go to the hospital," Reed responded, her tone increasingly defensive.

"Okay, for what reason, ma'am?" asked the dispatcher, for the third time.

"Hold on for just a minute and I'll find out for you," she said. Then remarkably, she placed the dispatcher on hold for forty-five critical seconds while the life of Christin Gilbert ebbed away.

Forty-five seconds is a long time during a medical emergency. It can literally mean the difference between life and death, but that wasn't the only delay caused by Reed's unwillingness to give the dispatcher the information he needed to properly respond to her call for help.

When she finally returned to the telephone, she was anything but helpful.

"Sir, I'm sorry, but I don't have that information," she said, her voice now laced with the clipped tone of annoyance. "All I know is that we need a transport to the hospital."

The dispatcher was incredulous. "So you have no information as to why?" he asked, now revealing a touch of annoyance of his own.

"No sir, I don't. I was asked to call," Reed brusquely replied. It was obvious that the walls had gone up, and she wasn't going to tell him anything.

"So do you need the police over there?" questioned the dispatcher. Suspicious, the dispatcher recorded that the caller was evasive.

"Oh, no, no, no!" Reed replied, as if the question were ludicrous.

"Well, that's why we ask these questions, so we know how to respond and what units to respond," explained the dispatcher. "If you can't give me that information—"

Reed didn't wait for him to finish. Indignant, Reed interrupted, "We just need a transport to the hospital."

The conversation was over. Not fully understanding the urgency of the situation, the emergency responders took nine long minutes to arrive at the abortion clinic. Once there, the urgency became all too clear.

According to information we obtained later, Christin was unconscious, with the abortionist on top of her, vainly attempting to revive her. Paramedics first thought he was a male nurse who may not have known what he was doing. EMTs were forced to pull him off and begin proper resuscitation procedures. Once they revived Christin, it took only four minutes for the ambulance to rush her to the Wesley emergency room, where Cheryl and Brenna were waiting.

Once we released the 911 recording, there was shock and outrage. Accusations began to fly, most of which originated from our flurry of press releases, that Reed's evasiveness and arrogant attitude may have delayed emergency help—a delay that could have cost Christin her life. Everyone from Governor Sebelius to the Kansas Legislature sat up and took notice. That recording was probably the single most damaging piece of evidence against Tiller's reputation, which had been stellar up to that point. There was little defense that could be made for such an obvious attempt to cover up the truth, especially by the only people that could have saved Christin's life.

The powers that be, whether it was Sebelius or Foulston—or both—knew they could never allow us to receive that kind of damaging information again. That was the first and last 911 recording we would ever receive in Wichita.

Later, as more ambulances came and went from Tiller's gate, the Office of Emergency Communications, under the direction of a particularly unpleasant woman named Diane Gage, became more and more hostile. One of our staff members was even threatened and escorted from the courthouse by security personnel after making a legal request for open documents related to a subsequent medical emergency at Tiller's abortion clinic. The blatant refusal to honor open records laws was appalling and illegal.

We filed a suit to force compliance, but the fix was already in. A hearing was held in which it appeared we would win in our efforts to compel Sedgwick County to honor the law, but the case suddenly took a bizarre twist. Ten minutes into the lunch break, the judge hunted down our attorney at the snack bar and ordered him to return to the courtroom. The judge immediately ruled against us and dismissed the case. So shocked was our attorney by this aberrant behavior that he was convinced a phone call had been made that ordered the judge to rule against us. The attorney was frightened by the implications and quit the case. We persuaded him to file an appeal to give us time to find another attorney, but no one else was interested. The case was dropped.

Today, we have found several excellent pro-life attorneys who understand the importance of information that can be gleaned from 911 calls placed by abortion clinics, but at the time, there was just no one who would handle these kinds of cases in Kansas. Those who protected abortionists took great pains to suppress the truth.

The abortion cartel understands all too well the importance of obtaining 911 calls and how damaging they can be. Today, because of our success in using 911 recordings to inflict damage on the abortion cartel, several municipalities are beginning to unlawfully deny requests for 911 records. We must fight to keep these records public so that abortion clinics can be held accountable.

If you want to create an abortion-free community, it is imperative to learn how to make requests for 911 records and understand what to do with them once you have them, as we will discuss later.

7

LA QUINTA INN SENDS TILLER PACKING

Have nothing to do with the fruitless deeds of darkness, but rather expose them.

—**EPHESIANS 5:11**

During that week of *Roe v. Wade* activities in 2005, when the death of Tiller's late-term abortion patient was weighing heavy on our hearts, we decided to launch a campaign to expose the participation of a local hotel in Tiller's late-term abortion operation.

Tiller used the La Quinta Inn on East Kellogg Drive to house his late-term abortion patients, who came to him from all over the world for abortions that were illegal elsewhere. The procedure involved a three- to five-day process that required patients to stay overnight. Without the facilities to keep the patients and their families at the clinic around the clock, Tiller made arrangements for his patients to receive a substantial 20 percent discount at the local hotel. In addition, Tiller weekly rented a room for members of his clinic staff who stayed at the hotel while late-term abortions were in progress, in the event of a situation that would require after-hours attention.

The arrangement was dangerous. Women were sent to the hotel after their babies were killed in utero. They were given powerful drugs that induced strong, sometimes violent uterine contractions, to be taken at the hotel without medical supervision. We heard rumors that women often delivered their dead babies in their rooms after hours before they could make arrangements to get to the clinic. Without proper emergency equipment or immediate access to emergency care, the hotel arrangement was not only inappropriate, but very unsafe.

We had carefully documented Tiller's use of the hotel over a period of months. We had pictures of Tiller's staff parked at his clinic and also at La Quinta Inn late in the evening. We had recorded conversations with hotel employees explaining the special discount offered to Tiller's late-term abortion patients. This was not just a casual business relationship. The hotel manager and employees went to great lengths to accommodate Tiller's needs, and rebuffed our efforts to persuade them to terminate their business relationship with Tiller out of concern for the women who were endangered by their arrangement.

So long had Tiller been using the La Quinta Inn as an integral part of his late-term abortion business that many thought that relationship would never end. We simply could not accept that defeatist attitude, especially since no significant effort had ever been made to persuade the hotel chain to break its relationship with Tiller.

Fueled by a string of documented medical emergencies from abortions at Women's Health Care Services, we fired off a complaint letter to the head of the national La Quinta Inns chain and then followed up with our *Roe* week press conference, protest, and press release calling for a national boycott of the hotel chain.

We were out before sunrise on Tuesday, January 18, 2005, braving the frigid morning temperatures while holding a variety of pro-life signs outside the La Quinta Inn. Images of babies aborted in the later terms of pregnancy were coupled with pronouncements that the hotel was collaborating in the carnage. All the while, our fleet of Truth Trucks circled the block, reminding motorists that a late-term abortion clinic was operating just down the street.

To the average passerby, the hotel was a seemingly unusual spot for a pro-life activity, especially at that early hour, but in this case our presence there served a twofold purpose. Housed inside were around ten women in the late terms of pregnancy who would soon be leaving the hotel to begin their three- to five-day late-term abortion process at George Tiller's infamous Women's Health Care Services. We hoped for an opportunity to reach out to these women and offer them abortion alternatives before they took that final drive down Kellogg Avenue with their growing babies still alive and thriving. We understood that later in the day, without our intervention, these women would receive the fatal injection that would cause "fetal demise," as Tiller called it, and then it would be too late for us to help.

Our second purpose was to draw public attention to La Quinta Inn's crucial role in Tiller's late-term abortion business. If we could only generate public pressure, we hoped La Quinta Inn would stop assisting Tiller, and perhaps that would negatively impact his business and save lives. Our early morning presence outside La Quinta Inn punctuated our press release calling for a nationwide boycott of the La Quinta franchise.

We are generally reluctant to call for national boycotts. If the corporation decides to ignore them, boycotts lead to failure and discouragement. However, Cheryl felt so strongly about this one that she went with her gut feeling. This time it paid off.

I was surprised when I was soon contacted directly by one of La Quinta Inn's corporate vice presidents who was horrified to learn how his Wichita franchise was being used by the most notorious abortionist in the nation. He assured me that the policy of using their hotel as an adjunct abortion clinic was finished.

On January 31, 2005, just thirteen days after we launched the boycott, a La Quinta Inn representative, Teresa Ferguson, informed me that Tiller was called by the La Quinta corporate office and told to immediately stop using their hotel as a working part of his abortion business, a practice they had determined was illegal.

Ferguson also told me that Tiller was advised he could no longer use the La Quinta Inn name to promote his abortion business and ordered Tiller to strip the name from all of his literature and website.

It was over. La Quinta Inns had sent Tiller packing.

We were exuberant and excited for the victory. While we understood that this was only one step toward our goal, what a giant stride it was! Newspapers across America published stories about the hotel ending its business relationship with Tiller. The longtime abortionist had to be demoralized by this very public defeat.

For the remainder of the years his clinic was open, Tiller bounced his patients from one hotel to another, never finding a long-term relationship with another hotel like the one he had once enjoyed. It created an inconvenience for him and prolonged the moral victory for us. To this day, some die-hard pro-life supporters still refuse to stay at La Quinta Inns because of one East Wichita hotel that enabled late-term abortions for so many years. Our thirteen-day boycott was a huge success.

Today, that hotel no longer exists at the corner of Rock and Kellogg. It was torn down to make way for highway expansion. The memory of its participation in the largest late-term abortion practice in the free world is all but forgotten by everyone but those of us who worked to expose its ungodly alliance. To us, the new businesses that now occupy that corner stand collectively as a landmark commemorating a victory that many thought was not possible to achieve.

8

LOBBYING 101

Politics is not a game. It is an earnest business. —**WINSTON CHURCHILL**

While the La Quinta drama was playing out, a bill, HB 2503, which would have licensed and regulated clinics that do abortion, was introduced in the Kansas House of Representatives. This law was desperately needed in Kansas since there was no clinic oversight mechanism whatsoever. We were convinced that if it passed, at least three of the seven abortion clinics operating in Kansas at that time would have been forced to close. The bill was strongly opposed by then governor Kathleen Sebelius and Tiller's now-defunct political action committee, ProKanDo. In fact, in previous years Sebelius had vetoed similar legislation.

Sebelius received large campaign contributions from Tiller and ProKanDo during her 2002 campaign for governor. During her time in the Kansas Legislature, she was known as both a staunch abortion defender and promoter.

As street activists, we had little experience with lobbying, but that didn't stop us from launching a massive—at least for our office—lobbying effort at that time. We needed to convince legislators, who had already experienced failure of similar legislation, to pass a clinic-licensing bill once again.

Cheryl led an all-women's press conference in the capitol rotunda supporting HB 2503. A former Tiller patient, Linda Cramer, told of her horrific experience at WHCS a number of years ago and of her inability to bear children since suffering abortion injuries. Cheryl discussed the death of Christin Gilbert. A legislator who was present at the press conference believed the statements would be beneficial to advancing the bill and asked them to testify before an upcoming Senate committee hearing.

After the news conference, Linda was improperly contacted by ProKanDo director Julie Burkhart, which Linda viewed as intimidation, to keep her from testifying. She was nervous and feared further repercussions from Tiller's bullies against her and her family, yet she was courageous enough to continue. On March 22, 2005, Cheryl and Linda testified before the Senate Public Health and Welfare Committee in support of HB 2503.

Afterward, we issued an e-mail containing the former Tiller patient's story along with her testimony. So powerful were the details of Linda's horrific abortion experience and the evidence of ongoing harm inflicted on women by late-term abortions, that the story gained traction and was distributed nationwide.

Today, we take excellent pro-life news services such as LifeNews.com and LifeSiteNews.com, and other Internet news sites, for granted. But in 2005, they were either in their infancy or simply did not exist. It is much easier now to get pro-life news and information to the masses than it was then. That is why the impact our story had was so remarkable.

Three days later, after our legislative testimony, Larry Buening issued a letter to Governor Sebelius with an "interim" report on Christin Gilbert's death. According to his report, the board's preliminary determination was that the care Christin had received "met the standard of accepted medical practices." Ironically, the autopsy report had not even been released yet, and no official cause of death had been determined!

"The Board is aware that office-based procedures and clinic licensure are currently being considered by the Legislature and wanted to provide you with an interim report," Buening noted. This telltale statement gave substance to our belief that Buening's correspondence was politically timed and motivated, and that his "interim report" was meant for two purposes: to derail the clinic licensing law and to protect Tiller.

We began to flood the legislature with e-mails and postcards bearing photos of Gilbert that we had found during that exhausting Internet search, and of ambulances carrying Tiller and his injured patients. We launched a phone campaign urging the passage of the clinic-licensing bill. People from all across the country made calls in support of the legislation.

While sitting in the balcony gallery at the statehouse during a debate, I noticed that some lawmakers had our website up on their laptops and were reading about Gilbert's death and the other medical emergencies we had documented. Finally, the vote was taken, and HB 2503 passed with a two-thirds majority in both houses, a feat that the local lobbyists claimed impossible.

Yet our jubilation over this improbable victory was short-lived. Sebelius later vetoed the bill, then applied political pressure to a number of the Democratic House members who had voted for it. When the override vote was taken, some of the House members flipped, causing the override to fail.

As disappointing as that was, our effort was not without fruit.

Everyone at the capitol knew that Tiller was hurting women and that his late-term abortion practices were suspect. Tiller was giving Kansas a bad name, and for anyone who may not understand the Sunflower State, that is the worst thing anyone could do. Once a respected member of the community, Tiller was fast becoming a pariah who was rapidly using up political capital he had carefully accrued over the years.

Finally, Christin Gilbert's autopsy report was released eight months after her death, a new stonewalling record for the state of Kansas. It determined that she had died "as a result of complications of a therapeutic abortion." The manner of her death was listed as "Natural," a determination that pro-abortion supporters and the media wrongly used to promote the false notion that no one was responsible for her death.

The report indicated that Gilbert had succumbed to a series of complications, including symptoms that fit the description of a condition known as *disseminated intravascular coagulation* (DIC), a rapidly spreading clotting disorder that can lead to massive hemorrhage and death. Also listed were the presence of bronchial pneumonia that Gilbert had developed during her multiday abortion procedure, and possible sepsis, a life-threatening infection of the blood. The autopsy report was devoid of any kind of plain language that could be understood by anyone outside the medical profession, and all mention of Tiller's clinic and the name of her abortionist were scrubbed from the sanitized report.

While this was meant to close the chapter on the topic, it was far from the last word on the tragic death of Christin Gilbert.

9

THE CITIZEN-CALLED GRAND JURY

"A grand jury would indict a ham sandwich, if that's what you wanted."

—NEW YORK STATE CHIEF JUDGE SOL WACHTLER, AS QUOTED IN *THE BONFIRE OF THE VANITIES*

Disappointment does not always mean discouragement, and while we were disappointed with the political interference in the KSBHA investigation and with the obfuscation of facts in Christin Gilbert's autopsy report, we were far from finished. We knew something else would come up to break the case open again, and as usual, it came in an unexpected way.

Cheryl had hosted a gathering of pro-life activists at her house for a meeting that was more focused on conservative political activism than on abortion. Yet, we understood that unless we changed the pro-abortion political climate in Kansas and voted out some of Sebelius's henchmen who were protecting the Kansas abortion cartel, we would never make much headway.

David Gittrich, the head of the Wichita office of Kansans for Life, was at that meeting. Seated on Cheryl's living room sofa, David broached the subject of gathering signatures for a citizen-called grand jury to look into any criminal culpability in the death of Christin Gilbert. Being from California, I did not know that such a thing was possible.

Kansas is one of six states, including Nebraska, North Dakota, Oklahoma, New Mexico, and Nevada, that allows citizens to petition the county for a grand jury investigation when the authorities won't take action on suspected criminal behavior. The process in Kansas involved gathering the signatures of a percentage of registered voters who had cast ballots in the last gubernatorial election in the county where the grand jury was to be convened. Those signatures had to be presented to the registrar of voters for verification, after which a judge was compelled to convene a grand jury to investigate the matters indicated on the petitions.

We discovered that we needed only a little over two thousand signatures to convene a grand jury in Sedgwick County. That was a very doable task. It could actually work!

Excitedly, we got down to the business of obtaining the required signatures on official petition sheets on street corners, at church meetings, and at any location where folks gathered. Then, in April 2006, we held a rally and press conference at the Sedgwick County Courthouse, where we presented our petitions calling for a grand jury investigation of George Tiller and Women's Health Care Services related to the death of Christin Gilbert.

We produced a video calling for justice for Christin that included the touching photos supplied to us by her grandmother. We had rigged the back of our Truth Truck with a projection screen custom made for that vehicle and projected the video onto the screen from inside the truck, to be viewed by rally participants. Every news station in town covered the event as we proudly picked up the boxes of petitions and walked them into the courthouse for presentation. Included with the petitions was a packet of information and evidence we wanted the grand jury to review. It gave them a starting point in their investigation of the Gilbert death.

On April 18, 2006, the commissioner of elections, Bill Gale, certified that 6,186 valid signatures had been verified, nearly three times the number we actually needed! The grand jury was convened and began its investigation on May 22, 2006. We hoped and prayed for indictments.

But on July 31, 2006, district attorney Nola Foulston released a terse statement announcing the conclusion of the grand jury:

> District Attorney Nola Tedesco Foulston announces that the grand jury impaneled to investigate the circumstances surrounding the death of 19 year-old [*sic*] Christin A. Gilbert on January 13, 2005 notified the Court today that it has concluded its investigation. The investigation resulted in no indictments being returned. The grand jury, which was convened in response to a citizen initiated [*sic*] petition drive, commenced its investigation on May 22. The grand jury performed its obligation in requesting and reviewing relevant evidence and law in the matter and has been discharged by Judge Richard Ballinger upon completion of its duty.
>
> The petition calling for the grand jury requested an investigation into alleged violations of the law, including but not limited to unintentional second degree [*sic*] murder, involuntary manslaughter, mistreatment of a dependent adult, and violations of the state's abortion and mandatory child abuse reporting laws.

(This press release can be seen at http://operationrescue.org/files/Grand%20Jury%20Release.pdf.)

I was livid. We quickly crafted a press release that screamed the headlines, "TILLER GETS AWAY WITH MURDER!" My statement in reaction to the unjust decision was brutally direct and conveyed my sense of outrage:

> We believe the lack of indictment by the Grand Jury is the result of corruption and cronyism at the local and state level. Nola Foulston is a personal friend of Tiller's and should never have been involved in the investigation in any way. The Kansas Board of Healing Arts, which earlier cleared Tiller in Christin's death is beholden to Gov. Kathleen Sebelius, who is in Tiller's pocket due to massive campaign contributions. We will continue to work to find avenues that are not corrupted by Tiller's blood money until Christin's killer is finally brought to justice.

Just days later, I received a call that changed everything. A prominent member of the grand jury had agreed to talk.

It was all very cloak-and-dagger. We met in the evening in a dimly lit corner booth of a local steak house. Cheryl pulled out her brand-new digital audio recorder purchased just for the occasion, turned it on, and plopped it down in the middle of the table; then the interview of our lives began.

Our informant was obviously nervous and did not want his identity revealed. He was not a pro-life activist by any means. He was just an average guy who ran an honest business in town, who just happened to have his name drawn at random from a pool of registered voters for grand jury service. I assured him he was doing the right thing and tried to make him as comfortable as possible.

He began to describe the grand jury process and discussed details of testimony that was given to him. So detailed were some of his descriptions that we knew he would have no way of knowing them outside the grand jury process.

The grand jury met for about three months and had access to a large number of documents in the case. The grand jury members also interviewed a number of witnesses, but were prevented from talking to some of the people most involved in Gilbert's death.

The grand jury investigation was limited in scope to investigating only the charges listed on the petition documents, and no more. The fact that a grand jury actually has the authority to investigate anything it wants once it is convened was kept from them.

During the interviewing process, a representative from the ambulance company was asked how many times, on average, the service was called to George Tiller's clinic.

"He said, 'Seven times,'" the grand jury member told us. "We asked, 'Seven times a year?' and he said, 'No, seven times a month.'"

We were stunned. We had documented only a very small fraction of life-threatening abortion injuries that had occurred at Tiller's notorious late-term abortion mill. What pro-life activists witness on the street outside of abortion clinics is just a peek through a keyhole at what really goes on. How many other women might have died and had their tragedies covered up? That is a question that haunts us today as much as it did then, because now we understand that concealing abortion complications and deaths continues to be "standard operating procedure" for abortion clinics everywhere.

The grand jury was not allowed to investigate the additional incidents that came to their attention. "We could only investigate what the petition asked for," our source told us.

We had been under the impression that the grand jury would have latitude to explore whatever they needed to. This was not how we were told grand juries work.

While district attorney Ann Swegle, who shared Foulston's pro-abortion ideology, behaved professionally, she appeared to be a neutral figure outside the investigation process, employing a hands-off approach to her interaction with the grand jury. Our source told us that "she was very articulate but not very personable. She was very good with putting things together, but we did not get the right information. She was totally out here [gesturing away from the group], and we were either going to figure it out ourselves or we were not going to figure it out."

Our source continued, "The DA wouldn't say anything unless we asked them stuff, because that's how it's set up. You [the grand jury member] are the investigator; they are there just to guide you. How do you know how to be guided if you don't know what to ask for?"

It did not take long for frustrations to arise as the jurors began their investigation.

Questions were raised as to how Christin, who had the mental capacity of a six-year-old, had become pregnant. Jurors were told that a grand jury investigation into that issue was ongoing in Christin's home state and would not be of concern to them. "That is a Texas matter, not a Kansas matter," the DA informed them.

While large numbers of documents and handwritten accounts were available to the grand jury, access to information from those most directly involved in Christin's death was denied.

A number of Tiller employees were called before the grand jury, but most "pleaded the Fifth Amendment," which prevented them from testifying. One exception was longtime Tiller associate Cathy Reavis, who was with Christin at La Quinta Inn the night before she died. Our informant said that Reavis spoke to the grand jury for about an hour and a half, but that she insisted she had overslept and was not present during the final episode with Christin at the abortion clinic the day she died. She gave them no helpful information when it came to uncovering what happened to Christin that morning.

However, Marguerite Reed, the receptionist who placed the 911 call on the morning of Christin's death, told the grand jury something quite different. Reed testified that she had met Reavis in a hallway during the forty-five seconds when she had placed the 911 dispatcher on hold. She said that Reavis told her she couldn't explain why, but that Reed just needed to get the ambulance.

Photographs taken at the clinic by pro-life sidewalk counselor Judi Weldy that morning clearly show Reavis's vehicle in the parking lot when the ambulance arrived at the clinic. Did Reavis commit perjury by lying to the grand jury about not being present at the clinic when Christin lay dying?

Our informant was disturbed by Reed's testimony and asked her, "Is there no sense of urgency? You guys are arguing about giving information to the people who are trying to help you."

Reed indicated that she never knew which employees were with Christin and had no idea what happened.

"We couldn't get any information out of anyone," said the source. "Without anybody speaking, we couldn't get any information out of nobody. These people can do what they want to, plead the Fifth, and walk. And I'm thinking, 'How stupid is this?'"

But our informant had another shocker for us. All the while we had assumed that Tiller had done Christin's abortion. After all, he had followed the ambulance to the hospital that day. But the grand jury member revealed to us that Nebraska abortionist LeRoy Carhart actually was responsible for Christin's abortion, and was "treating" her on the day of her death!

Carhart, a shoddy, late-term abortionist from Nebraska, was almost as well known as Tiller. He had defended the heinous practice of partial-birth abortion before the US Supreme Court twice, but his abortion mill in Bellevue, Nebraska, was a run-down, poorly maintained former car garage that looked as though it were one step shy of being condemned. The condition of his abortion clinic reflected his apparent attitude toward his medical practice.

Tiller posted calendars online that indicated which abortionist was on duty on any given day. Carhart's name appeared on dates when the majority of medical emergencies that we documented took place.

A subpoena for testimony was issued for Carhart, but on the day the grand jury convened to interview him, they were told by district attorney Ann Swegle that Carhart would not be available because he was in Nebraska.

The grand jury member elaborated:

> From questioning we found out the [doctor's] rotation from the "nurses" talking, and so the week he was scheduled to be here [in Wichita] we convened two days, and she [Swegle] was supposed to subpoena him. Well, he got smarter than us and he never came in. He was never served because he was never in the state.
>
> We couldn't subpoena him because he wouldn't come back into town. That's what the DA told us. Because he wasn't in the confines of the State of Kansas. He was in another state, Nebraska.

We knew that Tiller had been subpoenaed by a Texas grand jury investigating Christin's sexual assault. If the state of Texas could issue a subpoena to someone in Kansas, why couldn't Swegle subpoena Carhart in Nebraska? There was something very fishy about that. I sensed that the DA's office was obstructing the grand jury's investigation.

As the conversation with the grand jury member progressed into the evening, he gave us one revelation after another.

From the time Christin was brought to the clinic and "crashed" on the day she died until the time paramedics arrived forty to forty-five minutes later, there was an information blackout in records and testimony. Medical records provided to the grand jury were devoid of notations concerning Christin's care during this missing time.

"We couldn't get any information out of anyone," he said about the missing information. "We couldn't even find out who was back there" with Christin as she was being worked on for those undocumented minutes, but there were indications that unlicensed worker Edna Roach was assisting Carhart when Christin first "crashed."

When Roach appeared at the grand jury, she seemed arrogant and very unwilling to cooperate. She pleaded the Fifth Amendment to avoid giving testimony.

"Certainly not someone you'd like to invite to your Christmas party," he said of her. "Just a horrible disposition. She was just a very, very unpleasant lady. She was just blatantly laughing at the law. 'There's nothing you can do to touch me.' That was her attitude."

Witness after witness pleading the Fifth kept the grand jury from finding the truth.

Even a representative from the Kansas State Board of Healing Arts, the state agency that conducted an investigation that "cleared" Tiller of wrongdoing in Christin's death in late 2005, would not reveal what the board thought had transpired during those critical minutes.

Like Carhart, Tiller was able to avoid testifying before the grand jury. Tiller's legal team fully exploited a technicality in the law that threatened to draw out the process several months without any hope of getting any pertinent information out of him. This prospect did not appeal to the jurors. In the end, they gave up trying to interview him.

"George Tiller never showed his face," our source said. "He got his attorney to give us a little bylaw where he could go beyond pleading the Fifth, and it could stretch this thing out to up to eighteen months. We took a vote. If he did show up, would we ever get any information out of him? No. We chose to leave him still to be able to be charged instead of giving him immunity. The judge would not let us do that anyway. He said, 'I'm not—there's no way I'm giving him immunity.'"

The grand jury was flooded with medical and legal terms that they were not able, as laypeople, to adequately evaluate or process. "There are so many laws. We had all these laws being shoved right at us like we're in law school. We're just average Joes, and then if you want medical terms, I mean, there was just so much stuff to handle, which I think is ridiculous," our source lamented.

This hindered the jurors' ability to make an informed decision. The grand juror believed the grand jury should have been given more explanation and guidance concerning the technical legal and medical terms, and what their implications were.

In the end, the grand jurors sat down to make their determinations on the allegations before them. Some of the charges in the petition were discounted very quickly, among them the charge of second-degree murder.

"Second degree murder ain't gonna happen, and I'll tell you why based on very simply—nobody at that clinic intended to kill her. That's what it boils down to. If someone intended to do that, there was no way to prove, 'I'm out to get Christin,'" the grand juror explained. The vote on that charge was 15–0 against it.

In the end, the grand jury considered four counts of negligence.

First, they looked at the lack of education and training of Tiller's staff. Testimony was given that there were no licensed nurses employed by Tiller. His staff received only six weeks of training, after which he considered them to be competent to assist in complex and dangerous late-term abortion surgeries, even though the medical standards disagreed with this assessment.

Unfortunately, it was the grand jury members' understanding that Kansas law does not prohibit clinics from using untrained personnel. They were told that many clinics are set up this way. "If it's legal, it's legal," our source said, noting that such laws desperately needed to be changed.

Second, they looked at the way Christin was treated when she was brought in the day she crashed. The lack of notation in the medical records seemed problematic and prevented grand jury members from making informed decisions about the care she received.

Again, what the grand jury was led to believe—or allowed to believe based on a lack of explanation—just did not ring true to me. I knew of an abortionist in California who was disciplined by the medical board for doodling on a medical chart to the extent that his notations could not be read. But making no notations at all as to patient care during a fatal episode was just unbelievable. How could anyone think there was nothing wrong with that?

The third area of concern for the grand jury was the delay in placing the 911 call and the way the call took place. "They should have had her to the hospital immediately, not forty-five minutes later," the grand juror said.

Jury members were also concerned about Reed's evasiveness and the forty-five seconds that the emergency dispatcher was placed on hold. "I could walk a half a block in forty-five seconds. A minute could have saved somebody's life," our source told us.

Finally, the grand jury took a look at the "gray area" of time from when Christin entered the clinic on the day she died to when the paramedics arrived forty to forty-five minutes later. What happened to Christin during that time, and why was everyone involved pleading the Fifth Amendment?

The Fifth Amendment protects a person from giving testimony that may incriminate him. If there is no possibility of incrimination, there seems to be no good reason to plead the Fifth. An honest person with nothing to hide would just tell the truth. I was convinced more than ever that something illegal or unethical did indeed happen, and everyone involved was covering it up.

In order to issue an indictment, the votes of at least twelve of the fifteen jurors were required. Votes were taken on each of these four counts of negligence. Each vote was 11–4, one vote short of indictment. The same four jurors voted each time not to indict.

The problem seemed to be in the actual working of the negligence law. According to the grand juror, the law had two parts connected by the word *and*. An English expert was called in to explain the wording to the jurors. They were told that because of the word *and*, the action had to be both negligent *and* purposeful.

Because no one intended to kill Christin, the grand jurors who voted not to indict thought the negligence charge was problematic, in spite of the evidence. Too many questions remained about the quality of care she received, especially during the blackout minutes before the paramedics' arrival.

So, in other words, it wasn't enough that the clinic personnel were "bungling idiots" on the day Christin died, but they had to intend to be bungling idiots. All I could do was shake my head at the absurdity.

The grand juror's frustration was evident. The lack of testimony from those closest to the events surrounding Christin's death, the nonappearance of Tiller and Carhart, and the reticence of the Kansas State Board of Healing Arts to discuss the details of their investigation all worked together to prevent the grand jury from being able to adequately investigate and make informed determinations.

"How in the world can you ever find anything out when you can't get anyone to speak about it?" he asked.

Swegle told the grand jurors, "They can do that. That's how the process works."

"We were very frustrated to sit on that to try to make decisions on all the things the petition was asking for, and we couldn't make decisions because we couldn't get anyone involved to speak. We couldn't get anyone to say anything," the grand juror continued.

"So here we are trying to put this together. We're understanding what's going on here, but we can't make a judgment call when nobody has said anything to allow us to judge them."

The source concluded, "These laws, these things have to be changed, because all you're doing is letting these people walk."

We published a three-part exposé based on our interview with the grand jury juror, but it was completely ignored by the media. Tiller's lawyers complained long and hard about the "leaks" from the grand jury as if it were the worst crime ever committed. Of course, they would feel that way. The information that was brought to light was damaging to their client. All they could do to mitigate the damage was attack the messenger.

In the end, the dismissal of the grand jury without indictments left an unsettled feeling, not just among the pro-life activists of the state, but also among many in Kansas and across the nation who were following this case. Again, what was meant to "close the book" on allegations against Tiller only raised more questions and ensured that the final showdown was yet to come.

Later, a local pro-lifer group decided to launch a second petition drive to convene another grand jury, this time to investigate Tiller for committing illegal late-term abortions. We had deep misgivings that we attempted to address with one of their leaders.

The reason the first grand jury failed was because Foulston controlled the manner in which the grand jury was able to access and process information through her subordinate Ann Swegle. We firmly believed that as long as Foulston and Swegle had oversight of the grand jury proceedings, we could expect only the same results. A second grand jury under the same conditions as the first was an exercise in futility.

However, we were assured that the petition language demanded that an independent special prosecutor be appointed to direct the grand jury and that Foulston and her associates would be out of the picture. We reluctantly "went along," but invested less effort in the petition drive, which seemed to be acceptable to those local pro-lifers.

As predicted, the second grand jury was disbanded without issuing an indictment. The judge ignored the demand for a special prosecutor. Ann Swegle again directed this grand jury as she had done with the last. Once that happened, the outcome was inevitable.

This actually created another roadblock for us because it gave the Tiller side more "evidence" that our allegations were false and attorney general Phill Kline's investigation was nothing more than a "witch hunt." That was a club with which Tiller's attorney and the media would use to beat us time and time again.

10

BOUGHT AND CLOSED: CENTRAL WOMEN'S SERVICES

The gates of hell shall not prevail . . . —**MATTHEW 16:18 (KJV)**

While Tiller's abortion business was the focus of most of our attention, there was another seedy abortion clinic in Kansas. It was Central Women's Services, a run-down dump of an abortion mill on Central Avenue, only a block from Wesley Medical Center. An abortion business operating under a variety of names had occupied that single-story brick structure continuously since the first one opened there on August 31, 1983. It is estimated that as many as fifty thousand preborn babies were aborted there.

Once known as Wichita Family Planning, it was the site of some of the most dramatic and memorable rescues during the 1991 Summer of Mercy, including a Pastor's Rescue, where eighty-four clergy members were arrested on August 3 in what was said to be the largest incident of civil disobedience by pastors in US history.

During another rescue at the abortion clinic on Central, temperatures rose well over a hundred degrees. The pavement was hot enough to burn skin. The building was surrounded by praying Christians, who packed the driveway between the abortion clinic and the building next door. Police officers patrolled on horseback, their tempers as hot as the brutal Kansas sun. One of them lost control and drove his horse into the crowd of peaceful, praying families.

Jeff White, a California activist who served as tactical director for Operation Rescue, recalls picking up a large Gatorade bucket full of icy water and tossing it onto the blistering pavement, then ordering rescuers into the street to avoid being trampled by the charging police horses. The water cooled the surface enough to prevent the rescuers, most of whom were sitting in shorts, from suffering burns. Hundreds were arrested and placed in groups. Before some could be handcuffed, they crawled back to the rear clinic entrance on their hands and knees and had to be arrested again. Rescuers further delayed their departure in awaiting buses by doing what became known as the "Wichita Walk." Each rescuer in turn, who was asked to step onto the bus for transport to an awaiting staging location for processing, would comply by taking tiny baby steps. It would often take twenty minutes or more for a rescuer to travel just a few feet.

A dramatic picture ran in the *Wichita Eagle* that captured the horses stomping into the crowd. A large, framed color photograph of that same image now hangs proudly in our national headquarters as a testament to those who sacrificed their freedom to intervene on behalf of those being led away to slaughter.

But in late April 2006, Central Women's Services was on the ropes. I learned that they had not been able to pay their rent in months. Not wanting to lose more money, the property owners placed the building up for sale.

On the side, I often deal in real estate, sometimes buying and renting property and other times "flipping" houses to provide for the ever-expanding needs of my growing family. I had already purchased an empty lot directly across the back alley from the abortion clinic and placed a large billboard there warning women of the dangers of abortion. This sign faced the main entrance and was very effective. The clinic "escorts" hated the billboard and repeatedly vandalized it. The Truth Truck was also frequently parked in the lot during abortion days. After the property served no more use, I donated the lot to A Better Choice, the crisis pregnancy center next door. The lot has since been turned into a park.

It seemed logical to make an offer on the building when I found out it was being sold. I figured that if I owned the property, I could evict the abortion clinic and close it for good. It was a risky move, but with the encouragement of Cheryl and a very small number of other advisers, I made the decision to go for it.

I acted quickly to make an offer on the building through a third party. I did a little research on the owner and realized that he would probably resist selling it to Operation Rescue. Jeff White's daughter, Allyson, served as our representative and made an offer. It was accepted. The building was placed under contract and into escrow. Our contract specifically stipulated that the current tenant was not to be retained.

At that time, Central Women's Services was an open and functional, but unprofitable, abortion business. It struggled to keep an abortionist on staff. A series of abortionists drove down a couple of times a month from the Kansas City area about three hours away, since no one in Wichita would work there. Coupled with a dramatic 16 percent drop in Kansas abortions over the previous four years, it just wasn't enough to make ends meet.

Any company that loses 16 percent of its business is going to be hurting, and that might be truer for abortion businesses, which often operate on ever-shrinking profit margins. They don't have to lose 100 percent of their business before they close. Every baby we save represents a critical loss of income for many struggling abortion clinics that could eventually cause them to give up and close down.

While we had the building under contract, Central Women's Services somehow came up with the back rent and asked to continue their rental agreement with the new owner. However, because the property was under contract with the stipulation that the clinic would not be allowed to stay, the abortion mill was instead forced to close.

I have no doubt that if we had not moved quickly to buy that building, that abortion mill would have continued the killing for months, and might even still be open today.

In May 2006, while the building was under contract and in escrow, Central Women's Services conducted a yard sale. Everything left inside, including office supplies, equipment, and furniture, was up for sale. Cheryl attended the sale and was walked around the clinic by the former administrator—carefully avoiding the surgical area. She noted that the office was dingy, cramped, and dirty. There was really nothing of any value for sale. The decrepit furnishings were outdated and had certainly seen better days. The two plaid recliners that once occupied the recovery room caught her eye, but not in a good way. Like the rest of the office, they were filthy and more than a little creepy.

The abortion business vacated the mill immediately after the sale, leaving behind bad memories and the stench of death.

We were excited to get the keys and take the first real look at our new property. Jeff White joined Cheryl and me and our realtor on that initial walk-through of the vacant building. It was only then that the full scope of the filthy conditions was revealed.

The glass partition at the reception desk bore a sticker declaring that Central Women's Services had been a proud member of the National Abortion Federation and certified that it complied "with all the current standards of quality abortion care set forth in NAF's 2005

Clinical Policy Guidelines." We were about to find out firsthand what NAF's "standards of quality" really meant.

The carpets outside the abortion rooms were stained with blood, though it was evident that some effort had been made to clean them. The ceiling was broken and moldy. Toilets and other plumbing fixtures leaked. The walls were dingy, and some were covered with cheap contact paper that was bubbled and peeled. Dead roaches and mousetraps littered the floors, but it was the stench that struck us. It permeated every room. Bottles of OdoBan odor eliminator could be found everywhere, but they did little good.

A small closet between the two "procedure" rooms contained a sink surrounded by gallon bottles of bleach and drain cleaner. Under the sink where the suction machine bottles were washed was one of the biggest garbage disposals I have ever seen. The entire area reeked with the powerful stench of death. In fact, there were bloodstains around the metal band that surrounded the sink top. A bucket marked "biohazard" sat next to the sink. We were sickened by the thought of all those thousands of innocent children whose blood had been washed down that drain. It was an experience I will never forget.

During the initial walk-through of the building, we noticed that the phones were ringing. The abortion clinic had neglected to terminate their phone service. We spent the day answering phones and talking to abortion-minded women about the precious lives of their babies, and forwarded further calls to a local pregnancy help center where women received life-affirming information and counseling until the phone lines were disconnected about two weeks later.

After the tour of our new property, a woman approached our group in the parking lot to inquire about an abortion. Cheryl, a veteran sidewalk counselor, took the woman through the vacant abortion mill and pointed out the general filth inside the various rooms. The young woman was clearly horrified by what she saw. Cheryl continued to discuss motherhood and the blessing of children with her. The woman decided against abortion and left the scene with a commitment to keep her baby.

Since then the dozens of women who have come to that office seeking an abortion have been referred to the pregnancy help center next door, which reports 100 percent of the women referred to them from our building changed their minds about abortion. When abortion clinics close, lives are saved. It's as simple as that.

Mark Crutcher of Life Dynamics Inc. drove up from Texas with a cameraman to fully document the appalling condition of the clinic. We held a media event and allowed the public to view the video firsthand. I took the reporters on a guided tour. Most looked shocked at what they were seeing. Some covered their noses in disgust. But when the news reports were published, there was not one word about the clinic conditions! Instead, their stories were all about Jeff's daughter, Allyson White, and her part in helping us purchase the building years after her dad led those historic rescues there in 1991. Even after the abortion clinic's closure, the liberally bent local media still insisted upon "covering up" for it.

We finally began demolition on the interior of the building late in 2006. It was the first step of the renovation process. Nothing inside could be kept. The electrical system and plumbing had to be completely redone. We gutted the structure down to the concrete slab and cinder block, then sandblasted away the filth.

In January 2007, we held a ceremony at the building, dedicating it to the Lord's work. In attendance were many of the rescuers who had been arrested at that site during the 1991 Summer of Mercy for attempting to save babies from abortion. Rev. Dr. Gary Cass, founder and president of DefendChristians.org, officiated at the dedication ceremony.

The office was rebuilt with a new floor plan that included a large multipurpose meeting room that has been used for training sessions, press conferences, movie showings, and other public gatherings. Also featured in the building is a memorial wall dedicated to the pre-born as a reminder of the building's past as well as Operation Rescue's mission to stop the shedding of innocent blood.

Renovations were finally completed early in 2008, and we gratefully moved into our beautiful new national headquarters. The transformation from that filthy abortion mill was amazing! It was hard to believe it was the same building! Everything was new and geared toward saving lives.

This mill closed because Christians decided to take meaningful action. We didn't listen when we were told it couldn't be done. We stepped out in faith and let God work. The remarkable transformation of that building from a shoddy abortion clinic to a welcoming pro-life office that is closing abortion clinics is an *awesome* testimony to God's redemptive powers, and an example to others of what can be accomplished through faith, prayer, and a willingness to act.

11

THE ATTORNEY GENERAL INVESTIGATES

It is doubtful any criminal suspect in the history of this nation has ever so successfully used a high court to thwart legitimate investigations while persuading the judicial branch of government to put the prosecutor on trial.

—**TOM CONDIT, ATTORNEY FOR FORMER KANSAS ATTORNEY GENERAL PHILL KLINE**

Meanwhile, as the drama played out in Wichita, other efforts to bring Tiller and a Planned Parenthood abortion clinic to justice were under way in Topeka at the state attorney general's office.

In January 2003, a year after my arrival in Kansas, Phill Kline was sworn in as the state's new "Top Cop." He was soft-spoken, but a charismatic former state legislator with a deeply held Christian faith. He had promised during the election campaign to look into suspected illegal activity at abortion clinics.

It didn't take him long to make good on that campaign promise. In April of that year, Kline's office began an inquisition of Women's Health Care Services, Tiller's late-term abortion clinic in Wichita, and Comprehensive Health of Planned Parenthood, an abortion clinic in Overland Park—based on information he received that suggested the two clinics were failing to report suspected child sex abuse.

An *inquisition* is the official term for an attorney general's criminal investigation. While the abortion lobby used the term to invoke images of the Spanish Inquisition in an attempt to scare the public and turn public opinion against Kline, it was certainly more banal than that. Launching an official "inquisition" actually ensured that the investigation followed certain rules and safeguards, all under the oversight of a district court judge.

That investigation launched a decade of controversy and complex legal battles that continue to this day. There was no way for Phill, or any of us, to fully anticipate the force with which this investigation would be opposed, or the impact it would have on politics, policy, and the lives of those it touched.

The investigations began with a simple inquiry made by lead investigator Tom Williams to the Kansas Department of Social and Rehabilitation Services (SRS), concerning reports of sexual abuse involving children under sixteen. There was reason to believe that there would be few, if any, reports filed by Kansas abortion clinics.

SRS, under the political influence of the radically pro-abortion Sebelius administration, resisted providing the information and involving the coming weeks began to press the attorney general's office for the scope and details of their investigation. Kline believed that to inform them of details of an ongoing criminal investigation could compromise his office's ability to effectively determine the facts. In the end, SRS stopped cooperating.

The attorney general's office sought and obtained a subpoena for SRS child abuse reporting data through Richard Anderson, a district judge in Shawnee County, who would oversee Kline's abortion clinic inquisition. SRS grudgingly complied, sending Kline's office a confusing array of documents over the next four months. It took his staff months to make sense of the conflicting information provided.

In May 2004, Kline's office presented its findings to Judge Anderson, who ruled there was reasonable suspicion to believe that crimes had been committed. At Kline's request, Anderson issued a subpoena to the Sebelius-controlled Kansas Department of Health and Environment (KDHE) for Termination of Pregnancy (TOP) reports for abortions done from 2001 to 2004. Kline thought that a comparison of TOP reports to the numbers of reported incidents of child abuse might reveal whether the clinics were reporting as required by law.

KDHE resisted the subpoena, citing privacy concerns, even though the TOP records contained no patient names. Anderson rejected their baseless privacy arguments and compelled KDHE to produce the records, which would become a source of angst for years to come. KDHE finally released the TOP reports, and they revealed something no one quite expected. In 659 cases, the 2003 reports showed that abortions took place on children fifteen years of age and younger and/or involved abortions on fetuses more than twenty-two weeks old, which was illegal in Kansas at the time, with two exceptions. Such abortions could only be done if (1) continuation of the pregnancy would cost the life of the pregnant woman, or (2) the abortion would cause her a "substantial and irreversible impairment of a major bodily function" (K.S.A. 65-6703; see http://kansasstatutes.lesterama.org/Chapter_65/Article_67/65-6703.html). Kline was well aware of this law and its intent since he was serving in the state legislature at the time of its passage.

Based on the KDHE data, Kline's office began to actively investigate Kansas abortion clinics for criminal late-term abortions.

The Sebelius administration was aware that Kline's investigations were zeroing in on abortion providers, including Tiller, who were important campaign donors. Suddenly, the Center for Reproductive Rights (CRR) filed suit against Kline in federal court to challenge the state's mandatory child abuse reporting laws. Kline believed this suit was prompted by Sebelius in an effort to prevent the abortion clinic investigations from proceeding further. Federal judge Thomas Martin, an appointee of former president Bill Clinton, issued a temporary restraining order, also known as a TRO, preventing Kansas from enforcing its child rape reporting law.

Because of that restraining order, KDHE filed a motion to prevent Kline investigators from obtaining further information and seeking the return of the information already provided. This effort failed, and the CRR suit, derogatorily referred to by reporters as the "Kiss and Tell" suit, was eventually dismissed as moot after a minor change in the law, but not before the newspapers had publicly castigated Kline as a prudish man who was attempting to enforce his strict moral code instead of the laws. The stage was set for what would become an epic media character-assassination campaign against Kline, the likes of which have rarely been seen, even in the sordid history of American politics.

The next step in the investigation was to seek medical records from the abortion clinics, which likely contained more evidence of crimes related to late-term abortions and the underreporting of suspected child sex abuse. Kline had sought and obtained search warrants for the abortion records and asked Tom Williams to begin making preparations to serve the warrant on Tiller's abortion clinic in Wichita and the Planned Parenthood clinic in Overland Park. It is a matter of daily routine for law enforcement and prosecutors all over the country to request and obtain medical records as evidence, but there was nothing routine about this case.

After a discussion with his closest advisers, Kline reconsidered the search warrants and traded them in for subpoenas. I strongly believe that if he had served the warrants, history would have played out much differently than it did. Kline would have gotten the evidence he needed and would have had time in his term to properly prosecute. Perhaps that is a case of hindsight being 20/20, and maybe other events would have effected the same result. We may never know. But in the end, that one action taken early on in Kline's investigations ultimately doomed his efforts to hold abortion clinics accountable to the law and likely cost him his political career as well.

Tiller and Planned Parenthood resisted the subpoenas. After a flurry of legal motions, Judge Anderson ordered the clinics to comply. Instead, in October 2004 they filed a writ of mandamus under seal against Kline with the Kansas Supreme Court, using the pseudonyms Alpha and Beta clinics. This successfully allowed the clinics to delay compliance with the subpoenas pending the outcome of the secret supreme court action.

A *writ of mandamus* is an extraordinary legal measure whereby a higher authority orders an inferior authority to take action or stop taking action, depending on the circumstances, as required by law. In this case, the Kansas Supreme Court was asked to order the Kansas attorney general to halt his criminal investigation of abortion clinics and specifically drop his request for evidence contained in patient medical records due to trumped-up privacy concerns.

I had never heard of a writ of mandamus before. It seemed unbelievable that the subjects of a criminal investigation could sue an attorney general who was investigating them, and even more incredible that they could order the investigation dropped, especially after a district court judge had ruled there was probable cause that crimes had been committed.

Finally, about five months later, the case was unsealed and set for oral arguments on September 5, 2005. That must have sent the abortion clinics into a panic, realizing that the supreme court could potentially rule against them at that time and force them to hand the incriminating records over to Kline, who would no doubt charge them with crimes.

Two incidents then occurred that gave substance to concerns that the abortion businesses would go to any lengths to avoid compliance with Kline's subpoenas.

Just days away from a court appearance that could order them to surrender the subpoenaed abortion records, Planned Parenthood's Sheila Kostas requested information from Termination of Pregnancy forms that Planned Parenthood had submitted to KDHE from 2000 to 2004. E-mails obtained by our office showed that KDHE's Greg Crawford complied with Kostas's request the following day. This was an important discovery because apparently, Planned Parenthood had failed to maintain copies of the TOP forms in the patient files as the law required. If the files were subpoenaed as they were and the omission discovered, Planned Parenthood could face misdemeanor criminal charges for each missing form. Information supplied by Crawford could have easily been used by Planned Parenthood to fill out bogus TOP forms and insert the missing documents into the patient files to cover up the fact that they had not maintained the records as required by law. Did Planned Parenthood manufacture evidence to cover up crimes?

Then, on September 2, 2005, just six days away from the supreme court hearing regarding subpoenaed medical records, two huge trucks from a business called Security Shredding and Recycling Inc. pulled into the clinic parking lot of Tiller's Women's Health Care Services abortion clinic and began shredding box after box of what appeared to be medical records brought out by clinic and security company employees. The destruction went on for hours.

When asked about the shredding, Tiller's security guard, Carl Sweeney, flippantly replied, "Everybody's got to clean house."

One of our staff members photographed the incident, and we plastered it on the front of our website. We sent out a press release and tried to alert authorities that it was possible that Tiller was destroying evidence, but our concerns went unheeded. We may never know what was shredded that day, but along with Planned Parenthood's suspicious request for missing data from TOP forms, we could only suspect the worst.

Oral arguments in the mandamus case were finally heard, and the supreme court took the case under advisement.

Time moves at a painfully slower pace at the Kansas Supreme Court than it does for the rest of us. While the weeks slipped past, so did Kline's term in office. His 2006 reelection bid was soon in full swing. We understood that he desperately needed another term in office to be able to finish his investigations, file charges, and conduct a prosecution.

We weren't the only ones to recognize how critical the attorney general's campaign was. Governor Sebelius had handpicked Johnson County district attorney Paul Morrison to unseat Kline. Morrison and Sebelius's choice for the lieutenant governor post, Mark Parkinson, were both "moderate" Republicans who switched parties to run on Sebelius's Democratic pro-abortion slate.

In February 2006, the supreme court ruled that Kline was entitled to the ninety abortion clinic medical records that had been subpoenaed in 2004. However, the court constructed a bulky process whereby the clinics could redact the records, then produce the redacted copies to a court-appointed custodian, who would make further redactions. The process would prove to be laborious and time-consuming, but it was still a victory for Kline, although hardly anyone knew it.

We dropped a press release heralding the court's decision as a victory while at the same time the *Wichita Eagle* reported that the supreme court had ruled against Kline. It was perhaps the most egregious example of media bias ever. I have to wonder whether, if our press release hadn't revealed the truth, the editors would ever have recanted their false story. Eventually the papers were forced to acknowledge that the abortion clinics lost their bid to deprive Kline of subpoenaed evidence, but not without putting a negative spin on the story that would have given anyone vertigo.

"Kansas' Top Court Limits Abortion Record Search," shouted the *New York Times* headline on February 4, 2006, even though Kline was granted access to every file he had requested. The article then went on to imply that the court somehow viewed Kline as a danger to women's privacy, and as one who should not be trusted with unredacted medical files.

The article stated, "Before turning over the records, however, that [lower court] judge must re-evaluate whether Mr. Kline has sound legal reasons for seeking the records, the court ruled, and must eliminate from them information unrelated to possible violations of the state's laws on late-term abortions and reporting of child abuse" (Jodi Rudoren, http://www.nytimes.com/2006/02/04/national/04kansas.html).

The medical records issue became the weapon of choice that Kline's political opponents would use to wage a vicious war against him.

The political clash between Kline and Morrison was a battle of biblical proportions. It's hard to fathom anyone hating his political opponent more than Morrison hated Kline. The campaign was as personal as it was dirty. Over and over Morrison railed on Kline, belittling him for wanting to rummage willy-nilly through women's private medical records. Led by the *Kansas City Star*, winner of a pro-choice media award from Planned Parenthood just two years before, and its sister paper, the *Wichita Eagle*, the news media bolstered Morrison by maliciously attacking Kline at every turn. Editorials were written slamming Kline's abortion clinic investigations as "witch hunts." Their political cartoons depicted Kline as a buffoon. But the attacks weren't confined to the editorial pages. News articles were brazenly slanted and often reported information about Kline and his abortion clinic investigations that was just plain false. Little, if any, serious coverage was given to Kline's statements indicating he had never sought the names of adults who had received abortions, but only those of minors, so he could ascertain their safety.

To make matters worse, Tiller had dumped an estimated $1 million of his personal money into the race to defeat Kline. His political action committee churned out "educational mailings" by the ton, attacking Kline as "Snoop Dog" and scaring voters into thinking he wanted to post private abortion information on billboards around the state. Designating the mailers as "educational" allowed Tiller to sidestep campaign contribution limits. Things were not looking good for a Kline second term.

With only fourteen critical days remaining in his hotly contested reelection bid, Kline finally received the heavily redacted medical records three years after he asked for them and nearly nine months after the Kansas Supreme Court ruled that he was entitled to them.

Not to be deterred, WHCS and Planned Parenthood filed a second mandamus with the supreme court, demanding a halt to Kline's abortion clinic investigations fewer than twenty-four hours before Kansans took to the polls. That action was merely a political ploy for the purpose of further vilifying Kline in the final hours of the campaign, as evidenced by the court's wavering from its usual glacial pace to dismiss the case just a few days later.

As hysterical as the campaign rhetoric was throughout the attorney general's race, the people of Kansas allowed themselves to be manipulated by it. Kline was narrowly defeated by Morrison. He had just two months left in office. That would not be enough time to fully analyze the records.

In order to take office as attorney general, Morrison had to vacate his position as Johnson County district attorney before his term was up. Because Morrison had been elected as a Republican, the Johnson County Republican Party was entitled to appoint his successor. A meeting was held and a vote taken. They chose Phill Kline to replace Morrison and serve out the remaining two years of his term as district attorney in the same county where Planned Parenthood operated. This gave Kline jurisdiction to continue his investigations against Planned Parenthood and Tiller.

It was an unprecedented job swap, one that only intensified Morrison's acrimony toward Kline.

12

KLINE CHARGES TILLER

"You know, I've been covering the news in America for thirty years and this Kansas situation is the worst thing I've ever seen."

—**FOX NEWS HOST BILL O'REILLY**

Kline had just two months after he lost his reelection bid before he would need to leave the attorney general's office, and he seemed to make the most of them.

Kline's office analyzed the redacted medical records and found discrepancies. Every one of the records from Tiller's Women's Health Care Services showed that a mental health diagnosis was the basis for determining that the woman risked "substantial and irreversible impairment of a major bodily function" if her pregnancy continued. The law required a second physician unaffiliated with the abortionist to arrive at the same conclusion as the abortionist in order for the post-viability abortion to qualify for the narrow legal exceptions. In every case, the second physician who came to each mental health diagnosis was Ann Kristin Neuhaus.

Kline's office sent copies of the Tiller abortion records off for professional analysis to a distinguished Harvard-educated psychiatrist, Dr. Paul McHugh, who served as psychiatrist-in-chief at Johns Hopkins Hospital in Baltimore, Maryland, from 1975 to 2001. He was considered one of the most respected experts in the field of psychiatry in the United States.

I was contacted by an official in the attorney general's office, someone I cannot name due to a continued climate of political persecution that still exists in some sectors of Kansas, and was asked about Neuhaus.

We had thought that Neuhaus was out of the abortion business after she quit her part-time job doing abortions at Central Women's Services in 2001, and closed her full-time abortion clinic in Lawrence in 2002 after the Kansas Board of Healing Arts took disciplinary action against her for shoddy record keeping and abortion practices related to five patients. The board found she'd neglected to provide informed consent; failed to properly monitor the women before, during, and after the abortion; released them while they were still under sedation; and mishandled drugs kept at her clinic. In general, it was determined that her abortion practices presented a danger to the public.

In 1999, as Neuhaus was in the midst of her disciplinary case, she began "consulting" for Tiller, providing the necessary second opinion for his post-viability abortions. This arrangement began after Kansas Board of Healing Arts executive director, Larry Buening, called Tiller and recommended that he use Neuhaus for the sign-offs because she needed the money, even though he knew she was essentially incompetent. By 2001 she was the sole source of all late-term abortion second physician "referrals" for post-viability abortion at Women's Health Care Services.

We knew Neuhaus was the only "physician" working with Tiller to provide that second opinion, without which he could not legally continue doing late-term abortions in Kansas. She drove down on Mondays, interviewed the patients, then drove back to her home in rural Nortonville, about 175 miles away. We also knew that Neuhaus maintained no other office. She worked solely for Tiller at that time, and sometimes even drove one of his vehicles back and forth between her home and work in Wichita.

We filed a complaint with the Kansas Board of Healing Arts in October 2006 against Tiller and Neuhaus, alerting the board to what appeared to be an illegal affiliation between the two, and alleging that the post-viability abortions done with Neuhaus's help were in fact illegal. We had approached Kline about the possibility of charging Tiller under the illegal affiliation portion of the post-viability abortion restriction, but he assured us that his investigation was focusing on aspects of Tiller's practice that were more serious.

I provided my contact in the attorney general's office with Neuhaus's home address and the fact that we were aware that she stored her medical records at her home.

A subpoena was issued for Neuhaus, and on December 8, 2006, accompanied by an attorney, she submitted to an interview conducted by assistant attorney general Steve Maxwell. Later, we obtained a copy of the interview transcript. It showed that Neuhaus was hostile and uncooperative. Maxwell offered her an immunity deal in exchange for her testimony, but even then Neuhaus remained adversarial. Maxwell struggled to get answers to his questions but was able to wrangle enough out of her to confirm suspicions that Tiller had broken the law.

The AG's office finally heard from Dr. McHugh, their expert witness from Baltimore. He stated that Neuhaus's interviews were inadequate to conclude that any of the patients whose charts he examined suffered from any condition that would qualify for the legal standard of risking "substantial and irreversible impairment." Based on McHugh's professional analysis, there was only one conclusion. Every post-viability abortion done by Tiller and his three late-term abortionists had been done illegally.

On December 21, 2006, I was again approached by my contact in the attorney general's office. Before the news broke, I was told charges were about to be filed against Tiller. A group of attorneys were on their way to Wichita to file the papers, and they needed to know where he would be so he could be notified. I gathered my staff, and we spread out across the city, staking out places Tiller was known to frequent. I was excited at the thought that he would soon be placed in handcuffs and hauled off to jail, but as the hours ticked by, my hopes for such a dramatic event dimmed. As the business day ended without further word, we gave up our "stake-outs" and disappointedly returned home.

The next morning, the news was abuzz with the long-anticipated yet stunning news. Tiller had been criminally charged by Attorney General Kline!

We received a tip that Tiller's attorneys, Lee Thompson and Dan Monnat, would be holding a press conference at Thompson's downtown office. We hurried down to participate as members of the media.

Thompson confirmed that a summons had been issued to Tiller by a copy being placed in his door sometime overnight. He also indicated that he was in possession of the complaint, but declined to share the details with reporters because the case was allegedly under seal.

The press conference was a smoke-and-mirrors tactic to divert the media's attention while district attorney Nola Foulston was at the courthouse, finding a judge who would be willing to dismiss the charges. Foulston persuaded Judge Paul Clark to drop Kline's case on the dubious argument that Kline, the attorney general of the state of Kansas, had no jurisdiction to file criminal charges in Sedgwick County without her permission. Foulston denied ever giving Kline permission to file. The entire process took place in secret without proper notice to Kline's office.

Fewer than twenty-four hours after the long-awaited criminal abortion charges against Tiller were filed, the case was dismissed. We were as angry as we were disappointed.

Kline fought back. He released e-mails documenting that he had indeed met with Foulston before filing the charges and that she had agreed not to interfere. He got a new hearing before Judge Clark to reconsider the dismissal. We attended that hearing, again with high hopes, but the entire proceeding was a sham. Nola put on quite a show, prancing about the courtroom, waving various documents for emphasis. Assistant AG Steve Maxwell struggled to maintain focus on the true meaning of the law, but this was Nola's courtroom, where what she says "goes." Finally, the judge read his pre-written statement denying Kline's motion for reconsideration.

Knowing he had only a few days left in office, Kline appointed Wichita attorney Don McKinney as special prosecutor in the Tiller case. I considered Don a friend and knew him to be a dedicated pro-life Christian. He would often come out to Tiller's clinic and pray. In fact, he briefly represented one of my staff members, a young lady named Karen Myers, in a civil case against Sedgwick County. Karen had been jumped by two sheriff's deputies while we were picketing a concert put on by the radically pro-abortion entertainer Cher at the Kansas Coliseum in 2003. Karen was thrown to the ground and literally sat on by one deputy nearly twice her size, who continued to inflict injuries on her while he cuffed her for refusing to obey his unlawful order to disperse, which was in violation of our constitutional rights. The deputies falsely arrested me along with Karen. While I was being dragged off to jail, Karen's injuries were so serious an ambulance had to be called to transport her directly to the hospital. Eventually, the county settled the suit and paid Karen an undisclosed amount of money for the false arrest and her pain and suffering, which continue to haunt her to this day.

We had confidence that McKinney was not vulnerable to political pressure from the Sebelius administration and that he would be able to independently pursue a case against Tiller. On January 5, 2007, McKinney filed a mandamus with the Kansas Supreme Court, asking that Kline's thirty-count criminal case against Tiller be reinstated.

Foulston's arguments were ludicrous and grossly misstated the law. The chances of winning the appeal were great, barring any more corrupt political interference.

Three days later, Paul Morrison was sworn in as the new attorney general. The next day, he fired McKinney and announced his own "independent" investigation of Tiller. Morrison withdrew McKinney's mandamus before the supreme court could rule. Any hope of reinstating Kline's charges was over at that point, but we simply could not accept that. We were incensed at the injustice.

Providentially, we had an event planned just two weeks later that would bring national pro-life leaders and activists to Wichita, where we protested Foulston's corruption and demanded that the Kline charges against Tiller be prosecuted by her office.

Bill O'Reilly had been the inspiration for that event. The popular Fox News host had no love for late-term abortion. He often used cable television as a bully pulpit to denounce "Tiller the Baby Killer" and the horrific fact that for five thousand dollars, a woman could have her viable baby killed in Kansas, almost to the moment of birth, for any reason whatsoever.

During the "Talking Points Memo" segment in November 2006, O'Reilly spoke passionately against Tiller's late-term abortion business.

> Is this what we want in America? Is it? This is the kind of stuff that happened in Mao's China, Hitler's Germany, and Stalin's Russia. The American people cannot turn away from this—cannot ignore it. This kind of stuff simply cannot be tolerated in a civilized society. . .You know, I've been covering the news in America for 30 years and this Kansas situation is the worst thing I've ever seen . . . Americans cannot turn away from this; cannot ignore it. There should be thousands of people demonstrating outside Tiller's abortion clinic in Wichita.

We were not ones to let a golden opportunity like this pass us by! We are always looking at the national news for any way to benefit from it and use the attention a particular story garners to draw attention to our cause. If the Congress is debating the funding issue, we demand that they defund Planned Parenthood. If they are debating trade with China, we release a statement opposing any financial agreement until China halts forced abortions, their one-child policy, and other human rights abuses. The statement made by Bill O'Reilly during the most-watched cable television news program was tailor-made for us.

We immediately began plans for an event in January and called it "A Cry for Justice" and invited folks from across America to take up O'Reilly's challenge and come to Wichita. We quoted him at every opportunity. O'Reilly continued to hammer Tiller.

Just weeks before our event, on December 12, 2006, O'Reilly aired a powerful interview with a former Tiller patient, Kelly Stafford, who appeared on his prime-time show, *The O'Reilly Factor,* and told her graphic story of having had a late-term abortion at Tiller's clinic when she was just fourteen.

O'Reilly allowed Kelly to explain the abortion process in gruesome detail. She described how her baby was killed with an injection; then labor was induced. She was placed in a room with a row of beds containing about six other women who were also in labor.

"[Whe]n they decide that you're dilated enough. . . they put you in a wheelchair and wheel you out to another room. And in this other room there's basically a toilet," she explained. "And they told me to sit on the toilet, lean on the nurse, and push, push my baby into a toilet."

"What happened to the body?" O'Reilly asked Kelly, referring to the remains of her aborted baby.

"I have no idea. I left my baby dead in a toilet," she replied ("Dr. Tiller Abortion Patient Speaks Out!" partial transcript, Fox News, December 13, 2005, http://www.foxnews.com/story/2006/12/13/dr-tiller-abortion-patient-speaks-out/).

So powerful was Kelly's experience that O'Reilly struggled to maintain composure. He momentarily stumbled over words as he continued the interview. Kelly related how the abortion caused her to emotionally spin out of control until she eventually attempted suicide. Today, Kelly has recovered from her ordeal and has become a strong pro-life advocate who has accomplished much in exposing the horrors of late-term abortions.

After the interview, we were stunned! How could the rest of America not be?

Days later, the drama played out regarding Kline's charges against Tiller and the dismissal of the case by Tiller's friend, Nola Foulston.

Now our "Cry for Justice" event took on new meaning. Unfortunately, planning an event like that in the middle of winter is problematic, to say the least. January is not usually a time when people take vacations from work. The kids are in school. It's hard to get away. To make matters worse, in the middle of our event, a blizzard hit Wichita, dumping more than eight inches of snow and causing whiteout conditions throughout the Midwest. It killed travel plans for many activists. In the end instead of thousands, only a couple of hundred hardy souls showed up. Nevertheless, we protested Foulston outside her office and held a meeting at a local church to bring activists up to date on the status of the case.

The city had to plow out a space in front of the courthouse for our final pre-announced press conference. After trudging through drifts of knee-deep snow, I had just arrived at our newly shoveled spot in front of the Sedgwick County Courthouse when a man from Foulston's office approached and presented me with a letter from Nola. With interest, Dr. Gary Cass, Rev. Pat Mahoney, and Jeff White pressed in to peer over my shoulder as I read the letter, Foulston's response to our written request for a meeting to discuss our concerns.

"I find no reason to address these pending issues with you as suggested in your correspondence. You have been made aware that any attempt to influence this office and interfere with the administration of justice is criminal conduct," she wrote.

Wait a minute! I thought *she* was the one interfering with the administration of justice! And was she threatening us?

Foulston's letter continued, "The information that you have placed on your website, and your vituperative comments and continuous picketing will not influence any decision of this office."

Vituperative?! None of us had ever heard that word before, but it didn't sound very flattering! Foulston was digging in her heels, but so were we. Our press conference rhetoric was so "hot" it singed the ears off the reporters in spite of the arctic air temperatures.

Cheryl was anxious to release the letter, but I asked her to wait and let the lawyers deal with it. I don't think she has ever let me forget that mistake. We love our attorneys, but sometimes they take so long to do things that, too often, nothing ever gets done. That was the case here. We squandered a golden opportunity to expose Foulston for the corrupt and controlling dictator she was in Sedgwick County, who imposed her will and ideology with an iron fist—never mind the law! The law was just a tool to be twisted to her use.

Foulston couldn't deter us from pressing on. The story of Tiller's involvement in what we believed were illegal and dangerous late-term abortions was much bigger than a small-town district attorney, no matter how big her god complex. The overwhelming majority of people in America—around 90 percent—disapprove of late-term abortions and would like to see them abolished. It is the one subject on which the majority of pro-lifers and pro-choicers tend to agree. This story had captured the attention of the nation and had not yet reached its crescendo.

13

CRIMINAL CHARGES FROM AN UNLIKELY PROSECUTOR

On or about July 22, 2003 in the County of Sedgwick, State of Kansas, the defendant, GEORGE R. TILLER, did then and there, contrary to the statutes of the State of Kansas, unlawfully perform or induce an abortion on a 14 year-old pregnant female when the fetus was determined to be 26 weeks of gestation and viable.

—**COUNT TWO OF SEDGWICK COUNTY CASE NUMBER 07 CR 2112, *STATE OF KANSAS V. GEORGE R. TILLER***

Meanwhile, Morrison and Kline had traded offices and were adjusting to their new positions as attorney general and Johnson County district attorney respectively. Needless to say, the transition period prior to Morrison and Kline's job swap was marked by contention. Morrison's animosity for Kline spilled over to Kline's staff who were attempting to aid in his transition into the attorney general's office. At the same time, several former Morrison employees in the Johnson County DA's office had created a hostile atmosphere toward Kline and his team.

On the morning that both Morrison and Kline were to be sworn in to their new offices, Kline ordered the inquisition files transferred to himself at the district attorney's office. His trusted investigator, Tom Williams, made copies of everything and took them to Maxwell's home, where they were sorted in his garage, then delivered to those who needed them.

Williams asked a junior investigator, Jared Reed, to store the district attorney's copies in his apartment until they were called for by Kline. The Johnson County DA's office was considered so hostile that there was a very real concern that political enemies who worked there might attempt to sabotage the records and the criminal investigation. Reed was a young, single man who lived alone. The chances of anyone accessing the records in his locked apartment were practically nil. Yet the media and attorneys representing the abortion cartel seized on this as a means of attacking Kline for allegedly mishandling the records.

It was obvious that we had to keep up public pressure. One great way to do that was through a web-based petition. Operation Rescue joined with Women Influencing the Nation to launch such a petition at ChargeTiller.com. We gathered almost six thousand names and presented them to the Kansas Legislature, enlisting their help with pressuring Attorney General Morrison to charge Tiller, and it worked.

Two weeks later, the Kansas Legislature sent a letter to Morrison, asking him to reinstate the charges. Three days after that, the House Federal and State Affairs Committee passed a resolution that would have compelled Morrison to reinstate the Kline charges.

In order to engage the grass roots, we held a huge pro-life rally and press conference at the capitol, in conjunction with Kansans for Life, to support the House resolution. Attendees were supplied with bright red T-shirts emblazoned with the slogan "Charge Tiller" and encouraged to visit their elected representatives' offices before leaving for the day. The sea of "Charge Tiller" shirts washed like a red flood through the capitol halls.

Morrison was forced to respond. He sent a tersely worded letter to the House committee that passed the resolution that was reminiscent of Foulston's defiant missive issued just two months before.

"I sincerely appreciate your position regarding the thirty misdemeanor counts filed by the previous attorney general. Any further charges will be based on my professional judgment, not legislative action or political calculations," he wrote.

But there was more going on than his insolent letter betrayed. Morrison later told reporters that an announcement about whether or not charges would be filed against Tiller could be expected in "weeks."

This was enough to cause House Speaker Melvin Neufeld to blink. Even though he professed to be a pro-life supporter, he showed his true colors by blocking the resolution from a full house vote. Some of the pro-life legislators were incensed. Emotions ran so high that five members of the House Federal and State Affairs Committee, including the outspokenly pro-life Rep. Ben Hodges, tendered their resignations to the committee in protest of legislative inaction over the Tiller case. That bold action earned Hodges an appearance as honored guest on the Fox News show *The O'Reilly Factor*. Bill O'Reilly took the opportunity to lambaste Governor Sebelius as "not fit to serve" for her part in the Tiller late-term abortion scandal.

It didn't really matter that the legislature's attempts weren't completely successful. The petition generated public and legislative pressure that kept the case in the national public eye and brought down the "weight" of the state legislature on Morrison, making it harder for him to justify allowing Tiller to go scot-free.

About the time we thought that the situation couldn't get any more stressful, a bombshell development rocked Kansas.

The incident began as very cloak-and-dagger. I was out of town at the time, so Cheryl was secretly notified to meet at 7:00 a.m. in Overland Park in a shopping center parking lot from where she would be escorted to an undisclosed location. She had no idea why she was being summoned or what she would see at the clandestine meeting.

She met other Kansas pro-life leaders who had also received the same cryptic message. They were shuttled to a recording studio, where they met Jenn Giroux, then head of a group called Women Influencing a Nation. Jenn was a friend of Phill Kline's who was working to help get the word out about the political obstruction that Kline faced as he attempted to criminally prosecute George Tiller.

Jenn had seen a copy of the complaint filed by Kline and noticed a witness list for the prosecution attached to the back. That list contained the name of Dr. Paul McHugh, a name that had been previously known to us. He was Kline's expert witness who evaluated the abortion records obtained by his office through the infamous subpoena that prompted three years of legal wrangling by the abortionist under investigation. Jenn, a bold woman who wasn't afraid to make waves, reached out to Dr. McHugh, and he agreed to talk on tape. Since the criminal case he had been hired to participate in had been closed, there was no longer any reason for him to remain silent. She arranged to have him secretly flown out to Kansas and ushered to the recording studio.

A guard stood at the door as local radio personality Megan Mosak sat down on a professional studio set and began to interview Dr. McHugh. Jenn was concerned that if Morrison found out what they were doing, he would shut it down. At the time, Cheryl thought this concern was a bit paranoid, but later circumstances proved that Jenn was right.

Cheryl and other trusted pro-life leaders sat off camera, witnessing the powerful exchange, which was being captured on video. (You can view the full forty-four-minute video and read the transcript at http://www.operationrescue.org/noblog/fullmchughinterview/.)

Dr. McHugh indicated that he had been hired by then attorney general Phill Kline to examine abortion records and determine if the abortions were justified under the stated mental health determinations. He discussed the fact that after he submitted his affidavit containing his professional findings, he was never contacted by the attorney general's office again once Morrison assumed office.

Megan Mosak went on the record, asking Dr. McHugh specifically about his contact with Morrison's office.

"The new attorney general, Paul Morrison, he has stated that he is actively investigating Tiller and he even has an assistant attorney general on this case full-time. Has anyone from Mr. Morrison's office, or Mr. Morrison himself tried to contact you?" she asked.

"No, he hasn't," Dr. McHugh responded. "I expected I might hear from somebody. I never did."

Dr. McHugh had examined the records and made a number of professional determinations that were extremely damaging to Tiller and his world-renowned late-term abortion business. He stated that the abortion records contained inadequate information on which to make a proper psychiatric diagnosis and that he believed that Tiller's abortion clinic was misusing psychiatry to wrongly justify providing late-term abortions that would otherwise be illegal. Dr. McHugh noted that the late-term abortion justifications recorded in the heavily redacted abortion records were based more on societal issues than on firm psychiatric or mental health standards.

Dr. McHugh explained that the abortion records showed women who were twenty-six to thirty weeks into their pregnancies were being given abortions by Tiller for "trivial" birth control reasons under the guise of "mental health" concerns that could not be substantiated by the records. They "highlighted certain kinds of things, which . . . were sometimes of a most trivial sort, from saying that, 'I won't be able to go to concerts,' or 'I won't be able to take part in sports,' to more serious ones, such as, 'I don't want to give my child up for adoption.'"

Of Tiller's psychiatric diagnoses, Dr. McHugh added, "He had mostly social reasons for thinking that the late-term abortions were suitable. . . . Again, these ideas that he was suggesting—these were not psychiatric ideas; these were social ideas that he is proposing. And by the way, again, there was nothing to back these things up in a substantial way."

When asked if Dr. McHugh could find even one file that justified a late-term abortion by demonstrating that the woman would suffer substantial and irreversible harm, as required by Kansas law, he responded emphatically, "I saw no file that justified abortion on that basis."

In other words, the mental health excuses used to justify the late-term abortions under the legal exceptions were a fraud. Every late-term abortion committed by Tiller and his cohorts had been done illegally.

McHugh's words landed with the political explosiveness of a bombshell. We had to get this information out to the public. Immediately Jenn published a short video with excerpts of the interview on YouTube. Cheryl and others present were given a DVD containing the entire forty-four-minute interview.

The following evening, we had arranged for Dr. McHugh to appear before a town hall meeting and divulge his findings. For months, all the people of Kansas had heard about this was the incessant attacks on Kline and his investigations, which were regularly emblazoned on the pages of the *Wichita Eagle* and *Kansas City Star*. We hoped this would be the moment we finally broke through and could show people the truth.

Once at the hotel where the meeting was to be held, we noticed a man milling about the entrance and soon discovered that he was a criminal investigator with the attorney general's office. He was stopping all the older gentlemen and asking if they were Dr. McHugh. Eventually, he was successful at delivering a cease and desist order from Morrison demanding that Dr. McHugh not appear at the public meeting.

"Your statements to the media and to Operation Rescue and others regarding this investigation may well violate [the law] and threaten our ability to conduct a fair trial. Accordingly, you must cease and desist from your public comments, lest you be disqualified from appearing as a witness," the letter stated. (This letter can be viewed in full at http://www.wibw.com/home/headlines/7985772.html.)

Morrison then went on in the three-page missive to falsely accuse

Dr. McHugh of violating HIPAA privacy laws and engaging in a "politically-driven media campaign." In conduct unbecoming an attorney general, Morrison excoriated the good doctor, calling his actions a disservice to himself, Johns Hopkins, and his profession, and concluded by threatening to sue him to retrieve the five thousand dollars he was paid by the attorney general's office for his work.

Inside the meeting room, a standing-room-only crowd nervously waited for the meeting to begin. The air was filled with great expectation and anticipation. Finally, state representative Mary Pilcher-Cook, a trusted pro-life legislator, opened the meeting. She began by reading Morrison's letter to a stunned and angry audience after informing them that it was unknown if Dr. McHugh would appear due to Morrison's threats. WorldNetDaily columnist Jack Cashill cohosted the meeting and invited a number of legislators who were present to address the fidgety audience while awaiting word of Dr. McHugh's decision in light of Morrison's threats.

Finally, Dr. McHugh did arrive to an enthusiastic standing ovation, but informed the packed house that he would respect Morrison's request and refrain from making further statements.

While the disappointed crowd filed out of the hotel, we knew that Morrison's attempts to silence the truth were in vain. We uploaded the entire forty-four-minute interview in four parts onto YouTube and published a verbatim written transcript that remains accessible on our website to this day. The genie was out of the bottle.

The next night, Bill O'Reilly took to the airwaves with another segment about Tiller, focusing on Dr. McHugh's interview. He sent producer Jesse Watters to Wichita for a "gotcha" interview with Tiller. I helped Jesse locate Tiller gassing his armored Jeep at a QuikTrip near his abortion clinic. O'Reilly aired the tape of Watters surprising Tiller with questions about his late-term abortion business, and George responding by calling the police. The whole incident made Tiller look guilty as sin.

We followed up a few days later by publishing accounts that illustrated how late-term abortions are out of control in Kansas and that enforcement of the late-term abortion ban was nonexistent. One such story was about a healthy woman, with whom sidewalk counselors had spoken, who came to Tiller's to abort a healthy baby so as not to ruin her "tummy tuck." That woman went through with her abortion in Wichita despite having no risk of suffering a "substantial and irreversible impairment of a major bodily function." Women were getting late-term abortions of viable babies on a regular basis for appallingly frivolous reasons. Tiller and his staff were thumbing their noses at Kansas law.

Then on June 27, 2007, Morrison announced that he would not refile fifteen of the thirty charges brought by former attorney general Phill Kline that related to the misreporting of illegal late-term abortions. Morrison, who called the charges "ridiculous," stated that it was his position that Tiller could not be charged with criminal intent because he filled out the forms reporting late-term abortions the way the Kansas Department of Health and Environment required them to be filled out. What Morrison never addressed was that the KDHE was under the control of a political climate created by Gov. Kathleen Sebelius, who had rigged the system to emasculate the abortion age limit and reporting requirements in order to allow abortion on demand through all nine months of pregnancy for any reason whatsoever.

The next day, however, Morrison held a press conference where he announced the filing of nineteen criminal misdemeanor charges against Tiller for having committed post-viability abortions using business associate Ann Kristin Neuhaus as the second physician needed to verify that such abortions were medically necessary as defined by law. At that time, Kansas required that the second physician not be financially or legally affiliated with the abortionist.

Morrison also announced he would not reinstate Kline's fifteen more serious charges of illegal late abortions that failed to meet the narrow exceptions to a ban on post-viability abortions provided by law. Those charges, which had the best chance at obtaining a meaningful conviction, were gone forever.

14

THE WICHITA AWAKENING

To say that "prayer changes things" is not as close to the truth as saying, "prayer changes me and then I change things." God has established things so that prayer, on the basis of redemption, changes the way a person looks at things.

—**OSWALD CHAMBERS, *MY UTMOST FOR HIS HIGHEST***

In July 2007, we conducted a three-day event we called the Wichita Awakening in conjunction with the Christian Defense Coalition and the Cause to bathe in prayer the Tiller clinic and the efforts to bring him to justice. An estimated crowd of five hundred turned out for a candlelight prayer vigil outside George Tiller's infamous late-term abortion mill to kick off the Wichita Awakening on Saturday evening.

Rev. Rob Schenck led the group in prayer for an end to abortion. Rev. Pat Mahoney of the Christian Defense Coalition also addressed the group. Norma McCorvey, the now-repentant plaintiff in the *Roe v. Wade* case, who was known to the court only as Jane Roe, joined the throng of young people on her knees in prayer. As music played, the group surrounded the clinic, lifting their hands in prayer that the abortion clinic would close and that abortion would end.

Smaller groups gathered around those whose lives had been

impacted by abortion to pray for healing and restoration. It was a moving time of prayer. We knew God was listening.

On Monday and Tuesday, we conducted "Prayer Sieges" on the sidewalk surrounding Tiller's clinic. Hundreds of mostly young people from all over the nation wore red cloth tape printed with the word *LIFE* over their mouths as they prayed for an end to abortion, and that nineteen criminal charges filed against Tiller would stick.

About a dozen young people from a California youth group called the Survivors conducted a "die-in." With live Christian music playing on a sound system, the Survivors lay on the sidewalk, in the fetal position, surrounded by chalk lines such as would be seen around a body at a murder site. They covered themselves with red cloth to symbolize the innocent blood that is shed and to protest the killing of innocent pre-born children.

Each night we held outdoor rallies in a park located at the Mid-America All-Indian Center, where the iconic Keeper of the Plains, a sculpture of a Native American lifting his hands to the heavens, towered over Wichita.

As the sun sank over the Kansas prairie, the grassy glade at the confluence of the Arkansas and Little Arkansas rivers came to life with energetic praise and worship music and prayer that focused on repentance for the sin of abortion.

A group of nearly six hundred young people gathered to accept the challenge from Norma McCorvey that those born after the 1973 Supreme Court decision should partner with her pre-1973 generation to see an end to abortion.

Rev. Pat Mahoney shared that he believed God was ministering to him that we are in a time of breakthrough that would soon see an end to abortion. We prayed that Pat was right. We needed a breakthrough like never before.

15

COERCED ABORTION

The greatest destroyer of peace is abortion because if a mother can kill her own child, what is left for me to kill you and you to kill me? There is nothing between.

—**MOTHER TERESA**

Perhaps in answer to our prayers, public opinion against late-term abortions began to increase despite almost daily propaganda-like manipulations by the *Wichita Eagle* and the *Kansas City Star* to paint Tiller as a hero and late-term abortions as a medical necessity for women. In truth, there had never been even one reported abortion in the history of the state of Kansas that was done for the purpose of saving the life of a woman. Not ever.

An interim legislative hearing examining late-term abortions in Kansas was held in September 2007. This time, I was called on to present our documentation.

My PowerPoint presentation contained all our evidence of the many medical emergencies at Women's Health Care Services, complete with video clips and the Gilbert 911 recording. I made what I thought was a convincing case for the dangers of late-term abortion and the need for greater clinic oversight and accountability.

After my presentation, a woman came forward and gave bombshell testimony that stole the day's attention.

Michelle Armesto-Berge stood boldly before the committee with her attorney at her side and told her detailed shocking story of a coerced late-term abortion she was forced to endure at George Tiller's unaccountable late-term abortion clinic in May 2003.

Michelle was about to graduate from high school when she became pregnant by her boyfriend, whom she would later marry. Her parents were upset to learn of her pregnancy and immediately began to pressure her into an abortion that she didn't want. Michelle's boyfriend opposed the abortion, and together they had planned to marry and raise their child together.

Michelle's mother discovered George R. Tiller on the Internet and arranged for Michelle to have an abortion a few days later at twenty-six weeks into her pregnancy. After several days of nearly constant pressure and coercion, and fearing the loss of her family's love, Michelle relented to their demands.

Michelle and her mother became lost on the way to the abortion clinic and arrived two hours late for her appointment. Upon arrival, she was placed immediately into a group with several other women also receiving late-term abortions who were in the process of watching an introductory video of Tiller discussing his unique late-term process.

From there, without having spoken to anyone or signed any paperwork, Michelle was taken to a room with an ultrasound machine. The technician who did her ultrasound prevented Michelle from seeing the viewing screen. Then abortionist Shelley Sella came in and administered the injection meant to immediately kill the child through Michelle's abdomen into her baby's heart.

Sella is a California abortionist who once traveled to Wichita every third week to perform abortions at Women's Health Care Services.

She is perhaps most known for her work at another late-term abortion facility, Southwestern Women's Options in Albuquerque, New Mexico, and her part in the movie *After Tiller,* which debuted at the Sundance Film Festival in January 2013 and promoted third-trimester abortions.

After receiving the injection from Sella, Michelle was sent to the receptionist to fill out her paperwork and consent forms. There was no effort before the injection to ensure that Michelle was over eighteen, or that she suffered from any kind of condition that would meet the legal requirement of "substantial and irreversible impairment," either physically or mentally, for an abortion after twenty-two weeks. It seemed odd to her that she was not asked medical questions, but only questions of a social nature.

The next day it was discovered that Sella had failed to properly administer the fetal injection and that her baby was still alive. Michelle was forced to submit to a second injection procedure and was monitored until Sella was satisfied that this time she had successfully killed the baby in the womb.

No one offered to help Michelle avoid the abortion she never wanted while she was at the clinic, and one worker even went so far as to tell her that if she had the baby, her life would be over and that she would never be able to go to college.

Michelle delivered her dead child at the abortion clinic on the third day of the procedure. She refused to deliver her baby into a toilet bowl, as ordered by clinic workers. Instead she delivered her dead baby on the floor next to the commode, a sight that still haunts her to this day.

A minister from the Unity Church met with Michelle and told her that God would forgive her for her abortion, but he never asked her questions or even inquired about how she was doing.

Because Michelle's mother was set to graduate from college the following day, Michelle was released a day earlier than was normal, with the verbal promise that she would seek follow-up care in one week.

However, because of turmoil in her family and embarrassment over her abortion, she did not get follow-up care. She stated that Tiller's office never called her even to ask how she was or if she had indeed made the follow-up appointment.

Prior to her testimony before the legislative committee, Michelle requested her medical records from Women's Health Care Services and was shocked to learn that Sella had diagnosed her healthy twenty-six-week baby as "not viable" even though there was no medical basis for such an outrageous diagnosis. This designation allowed Tiller and his staff to illegally circumvent the Kansas ban on abortions of viable babies twenty-two weeks or older.

Michelle did not receive a second opinion as required by law for post-viability abortions at that time, and she was never diagnosed with any condition that would have met the legal standard of risking "substantial and irreversible impairment of a major bodily function" if her pregnancy had continued.

Michelle indicated that after reading the law that bans late-term abortions, she believes that the law failed to protect her and her baby from an unwanted abortion that has caused her painful consequences. She expressed that she is equally upset at her parents for pressuring her to abort, and Tiller for allowing the abortion to take place.

Every member of the committee seemed to be on the edge of their seats during Michelle's testimony. Rep. Jene Vickery noted that it seemed her abortion was done without any consideration of Kansas laws.

Nevertheless, the committee adjourned without taking action. A complaint filed on Michelle's behalf by Operation Rescue with the Kansas State Board of Healing Arts was quietly dropped by the board.

A legislative solution seemed like an unreachable dream rather than a sure reality.

16

MORRISON'S DISGRACE

And you may be sure that your sin will find you out. —**NUMBERS 32:23**

We were suspicious of Morrison's motives for charging Tiller and were concerned the charges were so weak that they would never hold up in court. However, we accepted the "gift horse" without looking too closely in his mouth. Thankfully, others did take a harder look, and what they found rocked Kansas politics to the core and changed the landscape of the Tiller case.

I received a late-evening phone call on Saturday, December 8, 2007, less than six months after Morrison had filed his nineteen-count criminal complaint against Tiller. An article by Tim Carpenter of the *Topeka Capital-Journal* had just posted online. All across Kansas phones began to ring, despite the late hour. Conservatives were getting each other out of bed to read Carpenter's explosive exposé. The next morning I called Cheryl and told her about it. As she read the account over morning breakfast, she called each new revelation to the attention of her husband with an excited, "Oh, my gosh! You just have to hear this!"

"Eye-popping" or "jaw-dropping" were common phrases used to describe the shocking details of the Carpenter piece.

An ethics complaint had been filed by a woman named Linda Carter, who had worked with Morrison during his tenure as Johnson County district attorney. That complaint was leaked to Carpenter through an unnamed source.

Carter alleged that she was in a sexual relationship with Morrison, a married man who was supposedly a staunch Catholic. Morrison and his wife even taught marriage classes at their home parish! During the bitter campaign against Kline, Morrison had boasted that he had not one hint of scandal during his administration as Johnson County district attorney. According to Carter, apparently that was simply not true. Their affair was famous with everyone who worked in the courthouse, the details of which were laid bare in Carpenter's lengthy article for all to see. (The article, titled "Sex scandal rocks A.G.," which we've quoted in this chapter, can still be seen on the *Capital-Journal*'s website, at http://cjonline.com/stories/120907/sta_224057474.shtml.)

But the affair was not the bombshell that jarred Kansans out of their beds that Saturday night.

According to the article, "Carter said in a signed statement that Morrison pressured her to make use of her position in the D.A.'s office to influence pending litigation involving Johnson County District Attorney Phill Kline."

Details emerged of Morrison's plot to leave his paramour planted in the Johnson County DA's office to spy on Kline's abortion clinic investigations. His plan was to use her to report back details to him so he could subvert Kline's efforts to bring abortionists to justice.

This wasn't just about sex. It was about corruption manifested in the perverted use of sex and power for political advantage. Morrison's obsessive desire to derail Kline's investigations through the sleaziest of means indicated not only critically impaired judgment, but conduct that was unquestionably unethical, immoral, and intolerable for a state's "Top Cop."

Morrison denied that he had ever attempted to coerce Carter into helping him derail the Kline abortion clinic investigations, but in light of Carter's detailed statement as reported by Carpenter, those denials lacked credibility.

Carter explained how Morrison pursued a romantic relationship, promoting her to positions so she could be closer to him. "Morrison made his feelings about Carter known to her for the first time while both were attending a June 2005 meeting in New York City," the article stated. Carpenter revealed that Carter was flattered but not interested. That didn't deter Morrison, who asked her to his room, where "he tried to kiss her. She rebuffed him."

While the public continued to view Morrison as a devout family man, he continued to pursue a sexual relationship with Carter. "I want to explore it," he told her, and the two began two months of flirting that eventually resulted in a sexual relationship initiated in an empty office of an assistant district attorney during business hours.

Carpenter's article detailed dates, times, and places of Morrison's sexual encounters with Carter over the following months as the couple shamelessly sought ways to use work hours and business trips to continue their affair. Carter signed for hotel rooms while Morrison paid for them in cash.

An appalling lack of discretion marked the relationship; nevertheless, Gov. Kathleen Sebelius rewarded Morrison's illicit lover with an ironic appointment to the new Interagency Council on Abuse, Neglect and Exploitation.

Carpenter left out none of the salacious details of Morrison and

Carter's business-hours dalliances. They "had sex in Carter's private office and in Morrison's office at the courthouse during normal business hours. . . . The two also had sex in a witness room assigned to District Court Judge Stephen Tatum," Carpenter wrote.

Judge Tatum would later be assigned to oversee a criminal prosecution of Planned Parenthood on 107 criminal counts filed by Kline as Johnson County district attorney. Tatum eventually dismissed the case at the request of Kline's successor, Steve Howe. Howe had been a longtime loyal employee of Morrison's with an axe to grind against Kline, who had fired him upon assuming duties as the Johnson County district attorney. Howe sued Kline for wrongful termination, but that suit was later dismissed. He later defeated Kline and took his place as JoCo DA.

Carter stated that Morrison had attempted to coerce her into signing statements that would favor Howe in his suit against Kline, but she refused.

Meanwhile, Morrison—with his wife at his side—continued to attack Kline's "lack of judgment" in pursuing abortion clinic investigations and his loss of "moral compass" for pointing out that Morrison had a documented history of sexual harassment. During this time, while he was taking the moral high ground in his campaign, Morrison's adulterous relationship with Carter deepened. He bought her "an engagement ring in December 2006" and gave it to Carter "during a trip to the Carter family's residence."

After Morrison defeated Kline, Carter thought she would be moving with him to the attorney general's office in Topeka. But Morrison had other plans for her. He intended to use her as his personal spy inside Kline's office. Yet, even that plan caused tensions between Morrison and Carter due to Morrison's hatred for and jealousy of Kline. "It was clear Morrison didn't want to turn over the keys to his office to Kline."

Nevertheless, Carter moved out of her home, left her husband, and took an apartment that Morrison frequently visited. Morrison had promised to divorce his wife and make a new life with her, but when it came time for him to tell his wife about the affair, he got cold feet. Carter was surprised and had even set a wedding date. Days later, Morrison rekindled his relationship with Carter, which became increasingly stormy, according to Carpenter's report.

> Morrison and Carter had an argument in March about Morrison's investigation of Wichita abortion doctor George Tiller. Kline had attempted to charge Tiller with violating the state's abortion statutes, but he was never was able to bring Tiller to trial.
>
> When Morrison became attorney general, he promised to conduct a complete, independent review of the Tiller case. Carter said in her statement that she urged Morrison to charge Tiller.
>
> She also said Morrison alleged Kline's approach to the abortion investigation was "unethical." The argument ended with Morrison storming out of Carter's apartment.

Eventually, Morrison did charge Tiller on nineteen misdemeanor charges after rejecting the stronger case filed by Kline. Upon announcing his charges against Tiller, Morrison shamelessly stated, "It was clear, after looking at the case, Kline's investigation of Dr. Tiller was not about enforcing the law. It was about pushing a political agenda."

In fact, Morrison's criminal case against Tiller was portrayed as technical violations that had nothing to do with the supposed quality of care provided by Tiller. From the onset, the case had little chance of success. Some even thought the case was intentionally weak to ensure that Tiller would be vindicated and Kline's investigations were further discredited. Others thought Morrison simply filed a weak case against Tiller to appease Carter, an allegation she vehemently denied under oath.

Morrison's relationship with Carter further deteriorated. Carter tried to sell the ring that Morrison gave her, but changed her mind and hid it in her apartment. Her husband, John, discovered the ring and sold it, putting the money in the family bank account. Morrison told Carter he wanted to have a baby with her, but then moved his belongings out of her apartment. Carter gave up on plans for marriage with Morrison and returned home to live once again with her husband, but Morrison again told Carter he wanted to marry her.

Through it all, Carpenter noted in his long narrative that Morrison continued to press Carter for information about Kline's abortion clinic investigations. He was particularly interested in how much Kline had paid expert witnesses in the case involving 107 criminal charges against the Planned Parenthood abortion clinic in Overland Park. Morrison had earlier cleared Planned Parenthood of any wrongdoing and appeared to be miffed that Kline was pursuing his own criminal case that Morrison could not block.

Morrison continued to profess his love for Carter as he pressured her for information about Kline's abortion case. To prove his devotion, Morrison got a heart-shaped tattoo containing her initials, but their frequent arguments became increasingly ugly. He called her a "monster" and "sociopath" and at one point threatened to derail her efforts to find a new job.

Soon after, Carter filed her sexual harassment case against Morrison with the Equal Employment Opportunity Commission. It was that complaint that precipitated the Carpenter exposé.

The Democratic Party in Kansas was stunned. Officials stumbled to articulate a response. At first Sebelius stood staunchly behind her handpicked attorney general, but within days, she threw him under the bus. Morrison was forced to resign in disgrace.

Operation Rescue was the first to call for Morrison's resignation. We celebrated and thanked God for bringing Morrison's secret sin to light and exposing the corruption in the attorney general's office that threatened efforts to bring Kansas abortionists to justice.

Morrison had been an unyielding roadblock to Kline's abortion clinic investigations, and we were ecstatic to have that obstruction cleared away. Kline's work, for which he paid a high personal price, appeared to be the best hope of getting the whole truth about Tiller and Planned Parenthood wrongdoing to the public.

Our celebrations were short-lived. Sebelius appointed former district court judge Steven Six to replace Morrison as attorney general. While Six kept a lower public profile than the gregarious Morrison, his pro-abortion bias was no less enthusiastic. When it came to thwarting abortion clinic cases, he simply picked up where his predecessor left off.

17

STEVE SIX

Corruption is like a ball of snow, once it's set a rolling it must increase.

—**CHARLES CALEB COLTON**

Newly minted attorney general Steve Six appointed Barry Disney to prosecute the Tiller case, which he had inherited from Morrison. Disney seemed like a stand-up guy, and we had hope that he would put aside the animosity Morrison had instilled in the attorney general's staff and try the case fairly.

That hope dimmed when I was personally told by an assistant attorney general under Six that the AG had told Disney not to take any "foul punches" against Tiller. In the end, Disney hardly took any punch at all. Before the trial he entered into a stipulated agreement about the so-called facts in the case, which greatly narrowed the focus of Disney's prosecution.

That stipulation allowed for only one of Neuhaus's letters of referral to Tiller noting that mental health risks presented a "substantial and irreversible impairment of a major bodily function" of the pregnant woman, and only one copy of her D-tree and GAF forms from one patient record. D-tree is a decision tool used to help guide better decision-making. In this case, a D-tree program used by Neuhaus was a training tool that asked a series of questions then computed a mental health diagnosis. The D-tree form was a computer printout that indicated the computed diagnosis. However, it appeared that Neuhaus improperly used the D-tree program to compute mental health diagnoses to justify late-term abortions and used the print-outs to document them in the patient medical record. "GAF" stands for Global Assessment of Functioning and uses a scale to determine how well a person is functioning in life. A GAF form would document GAF findings for patients' medical records. At the time of trial, we had no knowledge of the stipulation and had no idea what D-tree and GAF forms were. If we had, we would have cried foul from every rooftop.

The most devastating point to the stipulation agreement, however, was the following statement read to the jury:

> Before each of the abortions referred to in Counts 1–19 of the Complaint, Dr. Tiller determined that a continuation of the pregnancy would cause a substantial and irreversible impairment of a major bodily function of the pregnant woman, and that determination is not in dispute.
>
> Before each of the abortions referred to in Counts 1–19 of the Complaint, Dr. Neuhaus determined that a continuation of the pregnancy would cause a substantial and irreversible impairment of a major bodily function of the pregnant woman, and that determination is not in dispute.

That stipulation essentially told the jury, before a word of testimony was ever given, that Tiller did each late-term abortion for medically sound reasons in order to spare women from suffering serious irreversible harm from continuing their pregnancies. The text read as if it were a hard fact that these women's lives were in danger and that abortion was the accepted method of saving their lives.

Nothing could have been further from the truth! But the whole truth is something the jury would never hear, thanks to Disney's pretrial stipulation agreement.

While it was our opinion that Disney did the best he could at the time of trial under the restrictions placed on him, it is also our belief that Disney's hands were tied by Steve Six. We hope that Disney was no more complicit in this travesty than just following orders from his superiors. In the end, whether his involvement in covering the truth was overt or passive, it didn't really matter. That pretrial stipulation guaranteed the case's failure.

Later, Six inserted himself into another abortion-related case with national implications—one that cost him a seat on the Federal Court of Appeals.

In 2007, Kline filed a massive 107-count criminal case against Comprehensive Health of Planned Parenthood in Overland Park, Kansas, involving charges of illegal late-term abortions and manufacturing evidence to cover their crimes. The case was based on redacted abortion records obtained by Kline through subpoenas issued by Judge Richard Anderson while Kline was still the attorney general.

In January 2008, Judge Anderson gave testimony at a hearing in the Planned Parenthood case while Kline still served as Johnson County district attorney. He told the court of Kline coming to him with concern that records had perhaps been over-redacted, and that it was possible that some documents had been "manufactured."

Judge Anderson considered these concerns extremely serious and embarked on his own investigation, taking certain documents to a Topeka Police handwriting expert for analysis. There was a discrepancy, and Anderson immediately notified all parties involved.

"I had notified everyone that there was a questioned record," Anderson testified, according to a partial transcript reprinted in a later supreme court's opinion. "I had written a letter and . . . distributed it to Mr. Kline, Mr. Morrison, the disciplinary administrator, the Supreme Court Chief Justice, and said there's a problem with these records. I am going to sit tight. And I sat down like an old mule and just was going to sit on that until everything was cleared up" (*State of Kansas v. Comprehensive Health of Planned Parenthood of Kansas and Mid-Missouri, Inc.*, No. 100,726, Kans. Sup. Ct., http://www.kscourts.org/cases-and-opinions/opinions/SupCt/2010/20101015/100726.pdf).

Judge Anderson did indeed sit tight, but nothing was ever cleared up, thanks to Morrison's successor Steve Six.

In preparation for a preliminary hearing in the Planned Parenthood criminal case, Kline reissued subpoenas to Anderson and the Kansas Department of Health and Environment (KDHE). A motion to quash the subpoenas was held on April 3, 2008, and was taken under advisement. That same day, Steve Six, who was now the attorney general, heard about the possibility that evidence could be presented at a preliminary hearing on April 7, 2008, and immediately filed an emergency motion for a protective order with the Kansas Supreme Court.

However, Six withheld important information in his emergency filing. He neglected to tell the court that Anderson had previously testified at a hearing in January, where the "manufactured" records had been discussed. He also failed to mention that the preliminary hearing had been delayed six weeks.

Nevertheless, the supreme court issued a gag order on April 4, 2008, ordering Anderson not to testify or release any documents, while erroneously thinking that the information was still secret and that the preliminary hearing was only a couple of days away.

That gag order stood, delaying the prosecution of Planned Parenthood for over two years until October 2010, when the supreme court modified its order to allow Anderson to testify. The case went back to the Johnson County district attorney's office. There it was discovered that the evidence used as the basis for the Planned Parenthood charges had mysteriously gone missing. Howe concluded that it had been destroyed under Steve Six's administration as attorney general. He used the missing files as an excuse to drop the 107-count case against Planned Parenthood—thanks in large part to Steve Six.

Six was defeated for reelection by Republican Derek Schmidt, and the woman who had appointed him to the office of attorney general, Kathleen Sebelius, moved on to become President Barack Obama's secretary of Health and Human Services.

Obama would later nominate Six to serve as a Federal Appeals Court judge. That nomination was tanked by pro-life senators on the Judiciary Committee, to whom we fed documentation of Six's ties to the abortion cartel and his effort to thwart the prosecution of Planned Parenthood. After a contentious series of delays, Senate Judiciary Committee chair Patrick Leahy announced that Six's nomination would not be considered by the committee. As we like to say around our office, Steve Six's career as a federal court judge was "deep-sixed."

18

HIGH DRAMA

Questions are great, but only if you know the answers. If you ask questions and the answers surprise you, you look silly.

—**LAUREL K. HAMILTON,** ***BURNT OFFERINGS***

Before Tiller's trial, Sedgwick County District Court judge Clark Owens heard testimony during a four-day pretrial hearing in which Tiller's attorneys, Dan Monnat and Lee Thompson, put on a case for the suppression of evidence and the dismissal of charges. Monnat and Thompson had concocted their version of events that led to what they considered Tiller's unfounded political prosecution.

The hearing dragged out due to holiday delays that allowed for two days of testimony just before Thanksgiving in November 2008, with the final two days of testimony resuming in January 2009.

The casual observer might have thought the hearing was the trial of the century, as the courtroom was packed with mostly reporters, along with a few advocates on both sides of the abortion issue.

Several witnesses were called to testify, including Johnson County district attorney Phill Kline, who as attorney general had filed the original charges against Tiller that were soon dismissed by Sedgwick County district attorney Nola Foulston, a personal friend of Tiller's.

Defense attorney Dan Monnat engaged in the questioning of Kline that ran the gamut from boring and irrelevant to aggressive, offensive, and demeaning. Kline handled Monnat's often insulting questioning with grace, dignity, and sometimes humor that was lost on the dour Monnat.

In testimony perhaps not to Monnat's liking, Kline defended his investigations as being entirely an appropriate reaction to credible information received by his office that indicated abortion clinics in Kansas were failing to report child sex abuse. He subpoenaed records from the Kansas Department of Health and Environment that seemed to substantiate the information his office had received about the non-reporting. That led Kline to seek a subpoena from Shawnee County District Court judge Richard Anderson. The abortion clinics resisted the subpoena and secretly sued Kline to block his investigation.

After three years of legal wrangling, Kline finally prevailed and at last received redacted copies of abortion records from Tiller and Planned Parenthood just days before voters denied his bid for reelection as attorney general.

In an unusual move, Kline was appointed to serve out Morrison's remaining term as Johnson County district attorney. As he was leaving office as attorney general, he transferred his investigative files to himself in his new position as DA.

Kline revealed that in April 2006, he had gone to Shawnee County District Court judge Richard Anderson because he had reason to believe that abortion records he'd received through subpoena as attorney general contained evidence of a conspiracy between Tiller and Planned Parenthood to violate the Kansas late-term abortion law.

Nevertheless, Kline was ordered to return the Tiller records to then attorney general Morrison.

Kline said that he found that Planned Parenthood had referred three women to Tiller for late-term abortions even though the women were over the legal threshold of twenty-two weeks gestation, and that the women did not meet any of the exceptions to the Kansas ban on late-term abortions since they had no physical or mental health problems. Efforts to pursue that suspected conspiracy were blocked by Morrison.

However damaging Kline's testimony was to Tiller's dismissal motion, the star witness of the proceedings was Linda Carter, who was, of course, Morrison's former paramour. Carter alleged that Morrison had pressured her to interfere in a federal suit involving former attorney general and then Johnson County DA Phill Kline, and that he wanted her to gather information about Kline's abortion investigations for the purpose of impeding them.

Tiller attorney Dan Monnat posited the outrageous claim that it was Kline who had used the fear of the loss of her job to intimidate Carter into pressuring Morrison to charge Tiller. Carter adamantly and in the strongest terms testified that Kline did no such thing, and that he never discussed or hinted that he was aware that Carter was having an affair with Morrison until a month after the charges were filed.

Monnat's accusation against Kline was thoroughly shot down by Carter. Most of the questioning was just an attempt to smear Kline in front of the media. It was irrelevant to the criminal case against Tiller. Tiller's defense at that point was more about smoke and mirrors than about the real issues of law. It seems they hoped no one really noticed that it was Tiller—not Kline—who was charged with the crimes before the court.

Carter testified that she knew that attorney general Phill Kline had filed thirty criminal charges against Tiller related directly to illegal late-term abortions that were then dismissed at the request of

Sedgwick County district attorney Nola Foulston. Kline assumed the office of Johnson County district attorney and became Carter's boss after Morrison defeated Kline as attorney general.

Carter asked Kline to see the Tiller abortion records, copies of which Kline transferred to the district attorney's office when he made the transition from the attorney general's office. She said that Kline took the top three files out of a box of files and allowed her to examine them. Carter testified that it was part of her normal duties in the DA's office to review medical records and make recommendations as to whether criminal charges should be pursued.

After reviewing the records, it was Carter's opinion that Tiller had committed the crimes with which Kline had charged Tiller. "I saw the truth with my own two eyes," she testified. "I saw the records and made my own opinion."

Later, Carter said she and Morrison quarreled about the Tiller charges and Carter asked him, "Are you going to do the right thing and charge Tiller?" By that, she was referring to reinstating the thirty Kline charges against Tiller. She reemphasized that the question was hers and hers alone, and that Kline never suggested that she ask it.

As for Tiller's defense theory that she influenced Morrison to file the charges to please her, Carter told the court that Morrison's filing of the nineteen "technical" charges against Tiller made her "very unhappy," because she thought he should have instead reinstated the more serious Kline charges.

"I exerted no influence on him, and I don't think he considered my opinion whatsoever in filing the charges," she said. "It would have been futile on my part to try to persuade him."

Monnat violated the cardinal rule of witness examination: never ask a question for which you do not know the answer. Monnat was so convinced of his contrived conspiracy theory that the prospect that it simply wasn't true had never crossed his mind.

Judge Owens denied Tiller's motion for case dismissal, and a trial date was set for March. The ruling again thrust us onto that now-familiar roller coaster of emotions. At this point, anyway, our hopes were high once again.

19

THE TRIAL

A criminal trial is never about seeking justice for the victim. If it were, there could be only one verdict: guilty.

—**ALAN DERSHOWITZ**

When jury selection finally began on March 16, 2009, as always, Cheryl and I were in court. Our friend, Rev. Pat Mahoney, came from Washington, DC, to join us and led prayer meetings outside the courthouse every day throughout the trial.

Because Cheryl had attended every hearing in the months before the trial without fail, with me accompanying her most of the time, we built a great relationship with the bailiffs, which paid off in a big way during the trial.

Tiller's reputation was a national one, and his trial drew reporters from nearly every major news outlet. Satellite trucks lined the street outside the Sedgwick County Courthouse, creating a kind of circus atmosphere as reporters jockeyed for the optimum camera angle as they recited their stand-up reports live from the courthouse. In addition, there was understandably intense local interest in the case.

There couldn't have been a smaller courtroom in which to hold such a high-profile case. The gallery could accommodate maybe thirty people or so. Each morning a long line of folks waited to get a seat in the courtroom. The first day, we worried that there would be no room for us.

To my surprise, a bailiff with whom we were friendly came out of the courtroom before anyone was allowed in and called us over.

"You've been here for every hearing, and I'm going to make sure you get a seat every day," he said, then opened the door and let us into the courtroom first, ahead of the throng that had gathered. He even allowed us to bring Pat with us. Each day and after each break, the bailiff called us to select our seats first, before the public line was allowed in. We actually didn't feel too guilty about the special treatment because the public interest in the case was so great that it was streamed live on the Internet by local television stations. Anyone with an Internet connection could view the trial proceedings live on their computers at home or work.

Tiller received a jury of six with two alternates, who were seated during a routine three-day jury selection process called *voir dire*. Disappointingly, most of those who identified themselves as pro-life recused themselves from sitting on the jury, which left us with a predominantly pro-abortion jury. That decision of pro-life supporters seemed nonsensical to me. By walking away from that jury, they'd handed it over to those who held biases in favor of abortion. We need to stop thinking that because we are pro-life we cannot make sound judgments in legal cases! As Christians, we are honest people who are actually best qualified to fairly evaluate testimony and come to a decision on the facts of a case. I would have preferred that the Christians be dismissed by the attorneys or judge rather than for them to willingly walk away from their civic duty.

Finally, the trial actually began with high anticipation and a packed courtroom. Reporters were ushered into an overflow room where they observed proceedings over closed-circuit television.

The prosecution was up first, and now it was time to see what kind of man Barry Disney was.

Before testimony began, Judge Clark V. Owens II ruled on Disney's motion to disallow the proposed defense that Tiller was not responsible for violating the law since he consulted with his attorneys before hiring Ann Kristin Neuhaus, who provided all of Tiller's second physician referrals required for post-viability abortions in Kansas. The judge agreed that the defense was invalid and that he would likely sustain any objections Disney might make if that defense were used.

During opening arguments, Disney told the jury that Neuhaus was recruited by Tiller and trained by her attorneys. Tiller's attorneys prepared the referral letter that Neuhaus signed to rubber-stamp the late-term abortions. Neuhaus had no private practice in 2003, the time frame from which the charges arose. She saw patients whom Tiller and his staff had scheduled for post-viability abortions. She was paid in cash.

It was also revealed that in 1999, Tiller attempted to challenge the constitutionality of the requirement that the referring physician be licensed in Kansas. The Kansas State Board of Healing Arts had subpoenaed abortion records to ensure that he was in compliance. Rather than comply with the subpoena, Tiller considered filing a federal lawsuit to challenge the new interpretation of the law and thus avoid having to comply with the subpoena.

At that time, Tiller was allegedly contacted via telephone by Kansas Board of Healing Arts executive director Larry Buening, a longtime friend of Tiller's. Buening asked Tiller not to make a federal case out of this. As a solution, he suggested that Tiller make an "arrangement" with Neuhaus to provide his late-term referrals. Tiller immediately called Neuhaus and thus began their relationship. As soon as Tiller notified Buening that Neuhaus would be providing his late-term referrals from then on, Buening withdrew the subpoena.

Of course, Buening now denies that this conversation took place, but both Disney and defense attorney Dan Monnat spoke of that call as if it were what really happened.

Neuhaus was called as the prosecution's only witness. Her attitude under Disney's questioning was somewhat hostile. She lacked memory of any of the important points Disney tried to make. When she was reminded of her testimony under oath during a statement taken by then assistant attorney general Stephen Maxwell, she made excuses for the discrepancies by saying that she was defensive and felt attacked by Maxwell, and therefore she could not remember.

Disney had told the jurors that excuses are not a defense, and Neuhaus seemed to have unlimited excuses for not remembering anything. It was obvious that she was lying, which seemed problematic for her since she was promised immunity from prosecution only if she told the truth.

However, her memory seemed sharp when Tiller attorney Dan Monnat questioned her, and her attitude shifted to being much more cooperative.

At one point Disney took to the podium used by Monnat and told the court he would be asking his questions from there because the witness seemed more responsive to questions from that side of the room. The gallery laughed, but Neuhaus snarled, "Thanks for the smart remark."

Her attitude went from bad to worse. Her responses to Disney were argumentative and surly, prompting Disney to ask Judge Clark Owens to declare Neuhaus a hostile witness. After consultation over the noon hour, the judge granted Disney's request, but indicated her designation as a hostile witness would not be shared with the jury. Could that information have helped the jury understand the testimony better? Would it have made any difference in the trial's outcome? We will never know.

More sparks flew when Disney attempted to question Neuhaus about her discipline with the Kansas State Board of Healing Arts. Tiller's side strenuously objected—with good reason, considering her lengthy record of discipline—but the judge allowed the questioning.

In 1999, Neuhaus entered into a stipulated agreement with the KSBHA that limited her license due to finding that she had failed to keep proper drug logs or records of narcotics. She was ordered not to purchase any drugs other than valium or its equivalent, and was restricted from hiring anyone with a substance abuse problem.

In 2000, Neuhaus petitioned the board to amend her agreement to include the intravenously administered anesthetic ketamine, a request that apparently raised some eyebrows at the board. It noted that ketamine is not generally appropriate for use in adults due to the high incidence of psychomotor agitation and hallucinations.

The board interviewed Neuhaus about her request and found that she was not certified in advanced CPR, rarely inserted IVs in patients using conscious sedation, and, in fact, lacked adequate knowledge concerning sedation and relied on nurses to help her sedate patients. The board denied her request.

In 2001, the board found that Neuhaus had conducted an abortion on a sedated woman who indicated she did not want to go through with the procedure if it required that she be sedated. It also noted violations of the informed consent laws in other patients, along with shoddy record keeping. She was again placed on a limited license.

Disney did manage to establish through Neuhaus's testimony that she was recruited by Tiller, who consulted with her about the amount of her fee. He then set up a situation where she could see patients only at his request, at times that he determined, in an environment that he controlled. When she did the consultations by telephone, patients paid

Tiller's staff, and they held the cash for Neuhaus until the next time she came to the clinic. The form letter that she signed, referring patients to Tiller for late-term abortions, was drafted by Tiller's attorneys and provided to her by Tiller's staff.

Disney also established that patients were not free to choose their own second physician, and that Tiller controlled the fact that each patient saw Neuhaus, and only her.

After Neuhaus's testimony, the prosecution rested.

Tiller took the stand in his own defense and testified about his relationship to Neuhaus.

Tiller verified that on July 21, 1999, he received a call from Larry Buening, who was the executive director of the KSBHA at that time. He said that Buening told him, "Why don't you use Kris Neuhaus, and that will take care of all of your problems."

Tiller admitted that Buening told him not to quote him because he would deny the conversation. The only evidence that the conversation took place was a few scribbled notes in Tiller's organizational calendar. His notes indicated that Neuhaus was glad to do the consultations because she needed the money, something Neuhaus denied during her testimony.

Tiller's testimony under the questioning of his attorney, Dan Monnat, seemed well rehearsed and even memorized. But under cross-examination by assistant attorney general Barry Disney, Tiller appeared to have some difficulty processing the questions and giving extemporaneous responses.

During Disney's questioning, Tiller first indicated that he relied on what Buening told him as a representative of the KSBHA regarding the second physician law. However he later admitted that he did not exclusively rely on Buening's word in that 1999 conversation. In fact after the conversation, he told the court he still had questions about the non-affiliation language in the law and continued to consult with his attorneys about it for several more months. He filtered everything through his attorneys and ultimately relied solely on their advice.

In Kansas, claiming innocence because one relied on consultations with an attorney is not a valid defense against criminal charges, but that didn't stop him from trying.

Tiller admitted that his relationship with Neuhaus evolved over the first four years she worked with him.

At one point, Tiller began to refer to his relationship with Neuhaus saying, "When she was working for me," but quickly issued a correction stating, "when she was providing consultations for patients."

"When someone new was going to join your organization, it would take time [to set up]," Tiller stated, discussing the logistics of bringing Neuhaus on to provide the consultations needed for the late-term abortion patients.

In unguarded moments, Tiller revealed how he truly considered his relationship with Neuhaus. She was working for him.

Tiller further admitted that he profited financially by Neuhaus consulting with his patients. He estimated that he did 250 to 300 post-viability abortions in 2003, at an average cost of six thousand dollars each. He said that without Neuhaus's help, he would not have been able to do those abortions.

He told the court that his overhead is 62 percent of the fees generated by his clinic. His salary is 38 percent of the clinic's gross income. Tiller never said how much money he made from abortions prior to viability.

After crunching the numbers, we estimated that Tiller personally made at least $684,000 after expenses by killing viable babies in 2003, and we don't know how much he made killing non-viable babies because there were no numbers available. There was no doubt that abortion was a very profitable business for George Tiller.

The case finally went to the jury just before noon on Friday.

There were warnings that a huge spring blizzard was bearing down on Wichita, and meteorologists were telling citizens to hunker down for a big one. That was a bad thing for us. Convictions usually take longer than acquittals, and with everyone anxious to beat the storm and get home on a Friday, we were concerned.

After the jury went out, we left the courthouse and returned to our office. Before we could make plans for lunch, my cell phone rang. It was the sheriff deputy in charge of courthouse security. He notified me that the jury was in with a verdict.

We jumped into my Jeep and rushed to the courthouse. The big storm had begun, and already there was a four- to six-inch-thick layer of sleet on the street. My Jeep fishtailed down the road as I pressed the accelerator as hard as I dared. We ran in to the court. A deputy was holding the elevator for us. He shooed away others trying to reach the upper floors and escorted us past the line of people waiting for courtroom entry and into a nearby room, where we were searched and our personal property secured. Security was so tight that all anyone was allowed to take into the courtroom was a pen and a piece of paper. We were among the first ones seated inside the courtroom and sat nervously awaiting the long-anticipated verdict.

It was hard not to think of all the work and sacrifice it took to get to this point. If Tiller was convicted, it would be such an amazing victory, but if he was acquitted—I tried not to think too hard about that.

Finally, the jury was escorted in. The verdict was read. Tiller was not guilty on all charges. In the end, as someone said, the jury acquitted Tiller in less time than it took to eat a ham sandwich.

Attorneys for both sides went downstairs to the throng of media waiting in the courthouse lobby and made their statements to the press. There was certainly a mix of emotions. We knew that the case was weak, but we hoped that could have been overcome. It seemed as if it was back to "square one."

That's when we heard the news. The Kansas Board of Healing Arts had just issued a press statement of its own. It revealed that an eleven-count disciplinary petition was pending against Tiller, which would proceed in spite of the verdicts. That petition was based on Cheryl's complaint made three years earlier.

The roller coaster was headed back up the track. We were back in business.

We dropped press releases and made sure everyone who would listen knew that Tiller faced license revocation. The petition was based on the same patient files that were the basis for the criminal case. However, the Board of Healing Arts was concerned with the standard of care, and it had reason to believe that Tiller had breached that standard when doing late-term abortions in Kansas. We were excited about the prospect of getting a second chance to bring Tiller to justice. License revocation would be the ultimate victory.

Unfortunately, we would never get a chance to see it.

20

THE END OF THE TILLER ABORTION LEGACY

One who is injured ought not to return the injury, for on no account can it be right to do an injustice; and it is not right to return an injury, or to do evil to any man, however much we have suffered from him.

—**SOCRATES**

May 31, 2009, dawned as beautiful and warm for a Kansas spring Sunday as one could wish. I rounded up my bustling family and headed off, as usual, to Sunday services. With her husband at work, Cheryl enjoyed the peaceful, sunny morning outside on her back porch with a cup of freshly brewed coffee and a good book.

Then came the phone call that changed everything. I could hardly believe what I was hearing. George Tiller was dead!

As Tiller was serving as an usher and greeting his fellow members at Reformation Lutheran Church, someone had shot him in the head and fled. I immediately called Cheryl.

"How do you know this?" she kept asking, in shock from the news. I tried to get her to focus on the task at hand. We needed to put out a press statement with a condemnation of the murder and extending sympathy to the family.

Though the incident had just happened, news was spreading fast by word of mouth through this close-knit community. Phones were ringing all over the city. We didn't yet know all the details or who the suspect was, but we understood that people would want to hear from us.

We put out the following carefully worded and tasteful press statement, bearing in mind the need for sensitivity to the grieving Tiller family:

> Operation Rescue Denounces the Killing of Abortionist Tiller
>
> May 31, 2009
>
> Wichita, KS—It has been learned today that George Tiller was shot and killed while entering his church on Sunday morning, May 31.
>
> Operation Rescue releases the following statement:
>
> We are shocked at this morning's disturbing news that Mr. Tiller was gunned down. Operation Rescue has worked for years through peaceful, legal means, and through the proper channels to see him brought to justice. We denounce vigilantism and the cowardly act that took place this morning. We pray for Mr. Tiller's family that they will find comfort and healing that can only be found in Jesus Christ.

Then we waited to hear more. It wasn't long before our phones started ringing, and they didn't stop for weeks.

Our first call was from a reporter from whom we learned that the man suspected of killing Tiller was Scott Roeder. Scott was a quiet loner who lived somewhere in the Kansas City area and was primarily interested in attending any legal hearings related to abortionists. He had taken a particular interest in the Tiller case and phoned Cheryl from time to time to inquire about the date and time of court proceedings, as did many people during the trial. Cheryl's cell phone number was listed as the one to contact for information about our prayer vigils and other activities, so such calls were routine.

Nothing we knew about Roeder could have tipped us off to what he had planned, though Cheryl was uncomfortable with him for reasons she couldn't quite pinpoint. If there were two people standing in the hallway outside the courtroom, she would go talk to the other person and not him. He seemed to her to be a bit on the creepy side.

Imagine our shock and dismay when a news camera recording the towing of Roeder's car after his arrest zoomed in on a piece of paper lying on the dashboard, which read, "Op Rescue Cheryl" and below it her cell phone number.

Instantly, Cheryl began receiving death threats literally by the hundreds. No one bothered to find out why Roeder had her number. It was just assumed that she was part of a conspiracy to murder Tiller, when in reality nothing could have been further from the truth. To this day, she still has to endure false accusations from radical pro-abortionists who routinely take to the Internet to spread their slander concerning her fictitious involvement in Tiller's death.

My cell phone as well as the office phones received hundreds of calls and voice mails with additional threats to our and our families' lives. Our website was inundated and crashed. It was a frightening time. We stopped all interviews and tried to let sanity prevail. We closed the office for a few days in the interest of safety.

After a few trying days, our website was restored and we began posting stories unrelated to Tiller's murder. We tried to continue with "business as usual," even though much of my time was spent on the phone with attorneys in the event we were questioned.

We never were. In fact, we were contacted by the Wichita Police Department out of concern for our safety. We were given tips on how to improve our security, and a phone number to call if we had any concerns.

Soon after Tiller died, we received some shocking news. We were told that Tiller had announced his retirement to his employees just two weeks before his murder. That news was confirmed by LeRoy Carhart, who made public statements about Tiller's retirement announcement during public appearances. Unbeknownst to us, Tiller had planned to close his clinic for good.

We had noticed changes in Tiller's operation in the weeks before his passing. He closed down his political action committee, and his hired lobbyist moved away. Edna Roach, who had worked for Tiller for many years, had quit. Another longtime employee, Sara Love, stopped at the gate the Friday before Tiller was killed and told sidewalk counselors it was her last day on the job. The news that Tiller had planned to retire made all those curious incidents make sense.

What would prompt this decision by Tiller, who had fought for decades to keep his clinic open? The answer can be found in the insights of his close associate Shelley Sella, who shared in an interview with MSNBC Tiller's reaction to the Kansas Board of Healing Arts disciplinary petition that was announced immediately after his acquittal on criminal charges. That petition was based on one of our complaints. Of that petition she stated, "Why? Because one of the Operation Rescue people lodged a complaint on the same charges. He didn't even have time to enjoy the fact that he had finally won. And then, another blow. It was just never going to end." (The interview was aired October 25, 2010, in the special report "The Assassination of Dr. Tiller.")

Retirement was one way to make it end, and that was the route he planned to take. If it had not been for Scott Roeder, we could have publicly accepted Tiller's unconditional surrender and used that victory to encourage and reenergize the pro-life movement. Instead, Tiller's murder sadly snatched defeat from the mouth of victory.

Slowly, the uproar over Tiller's murder began to die down. We are thankful that Roeder was eventually convicted and packed off to begin serving a life sentence without the possibility of parole, closing that traumatic chapter for good. Sella and Robinson moved the remnants of Tiller's late-term abortion business to Albuquerque, New Mexico, a liberal Western enclave with virtually no abortion laws, as I believe was Tiller's plan all along.

We made a conscious effort to move on. We conducted a website upgrade with a new look and began to move the focus of our work away from Kansas. Suddenly, we had more time for projects that had been back-burnered by the frenetic pace of the Tiller project.

Our experiences in California and Kansas had prepared us for the next phase of our lives as pro-life activists. It was only after our Kansas project was concluded that Operation Rescue began to grow in influence and reputation through the exposure of abortionists around the nation who were breaking the law. We were suddenly seeing abortion clinics close and abortionists disciplined because of our work around the country. It was the kind of work that no one else was doing at that time. Our work flourished. Sometimes God has a way of moving us on through traumatic events into a new place where He wants us to be, and we were now exactly where He wanted us.

Today, Kansas is a very different place than it was when we moved from Southern California's pinewood mountains around Lake Arrowhead and the sunny shores of San Diego to take on a new challenge inside the boxy borders of the Sunflower State.

Tiller's political action committee disbanded in early 2009, just months before Tiller's unfortunate death.

Without Tiller's millions being pumped into the campaigns, Republicans swept into the governor's mansion and every other state office during the 2010 midterm election. A few months later, a clinic-licensing bill very similar to HB 2503 was passed and signed into law by pro-life governor Sam Brownback.

Slowly but surely, the old Sebelius-era cronies were purged from state agencies. Buening was replaced at the Board of Healing Arts, with which we now have an excellent working relationship. The Kansas Department of Health and Environment no longer coaches abortionists on how to slip through the loopholes of the law. Even Nola Foulston retired as Sedgwick County district attorney.

Since Tiller's death there have been efforts—mostly by those who live outside Kansas—to paint Tiller as a hero, but to do so they had to remake his public image. Before his murder, Tiller's official mug shot often stood as a backdrop to evening news stories concerning America's most notorious late-term abortionist. Today, we see only a "glamour shot" of an airbrushed man pictured in diffused light that lends an almost saintly quality to his portrait.

Months later, a story in *GQ* put it this way:

> But George Tiller is dead, and speaking of the dead makes people careful. But, also, because by now the small community of people around George Tiller knew the first rule was to deny the enemy any source material.
>
> Once they got their hands on something, they could do anything they wanted with it. They could isolate a quote like a strand of DNA and then make up a whole new organism around it. George Tiller's friends knew that one of their jobs was to protect him, in death as in life. [Devin Friedman, "Savior vs. Savior," GQ, February 2010, http://www.gq.com/news-politics/big-issues/201002/abortion-debate-george-tiller-scott-roeder?currentPage=1]

And so began the remaking of the image of the man known around the world as "Tiller the Killer."

But the reality of who George Tiller was—at least professionally—comes in the anguished stories of women and families who made the mistake of seeking out his unique services for three decades in the nondescript beige building on the corner of Kellogg and Bleckley in this Midwestern community tucked away on the southern Kansas prairie.

Tiller was no hero to those women.

There was the adoptive family of Baby Sarah, who was delivered in the parking lot of a local hospital after Tiller botched an attempted late-term abortion in 1993. He had attempted to inject Sarah's heart with potassium chloride to begin the abortion, but the baby turned, and he injected her in the nape of the neck instead. Although doctors said Sarah would not survive eight weeks, under the loving care of her new family she lived for five years. Tiller's attack on Sarah impaired her growth and left her brain damaged, blind, and unable to walk. A family member noted at her memorial service that Tiller succeeded in killing little Sarah, but it took him five years to do it.

The family of a baby girl we call "Baby Chelsea" had no kind words for Tiller once the reality of what he had done to their daughter sank in. Having received the diagnosis of cystic fibrosis for their pre-born baby, Chelsea's young parents heeded their doctor's advice and visited Tiller's abortion clinic in 1998. Chelsea's tiny heart was injected with poison, and she was delivered feet first. Tiller punctured the base of Chelsea's skull and evacuated the contents. Her head collapsed and slid from the birth canal.

Following the abortion, George Tiller baptized Chelsea, wrapped her in a blanket, and presented her to her parents for viewing, commenting, "Your baby was a very efficient parasite." Tiller then snapped Polaroid photos of the parents and their dead child, which now are carefully tucked away in a photo album cherished by a regretful mother. As she held her baby's body, fluids and blood from the incision at the base of the skull began to leak down her arm. "I felt like my life was draining down my arm," she remarked later. The abortion of her daughter continues to haunt Chelsea's mother today.

And who can forget Christin A. Gilbert, who walked into Tiller's abortion clinic, but was carried out on a gurney? Certainly Tiller was no hero to those who grieved her tragic and avoidable death.

Michelle Armesto-Berge, whose story we told in chapter 15, will never be the same since her appalling late-term abortion experience at Tiller's abortion clinic in 2003. Her abortion strained her relationship with her parents and inflicted emotional pain of a kind that only those who have lost a beloved child might be able to comprehend.

Then there was the woman we call Patient S., who was willing to tell us her story from her hospital bed. Patient S. sought an abortion from Tiller in September 2008. It was almost the last thing she ever did.

At the clinic, she developed a fever of 104 degrees and was held in a room, sick and without care, against her will for four hours. Tiller attempted to send her away—even though her abortion was in progress—when she expressed displeasure with the way she was being treated. When the abortion was finally completed, she suffered respiratory and cardiac arrest. She also developed an infection from a dirty oxygen mask used during the medical emergency. After being revived, Patient S. was taken to the hospital in Tiller's private vehicle and was told to keep her IV bag down so protesters would not see it. To add to the emotional pain, she felt her baby move just before the abortion and was convinced that her baby was alive.

Tiller wasn't much of a hero to those women, either.

Things were beginning to change in America even before the passing of the nation's most infamous abortionist. The pro-life movement was making giant leaps toward correcting the faulty public perception that abortionists were victims and the pro-lifers were the villains. Pro-life sentiment was beginning to rise in the polls. Just days before Tiller's death, a Gallup poll indicated that the percentage of Americans self-identifying as pro-life overtook pro-choice support for the first time in fifteen years. Americans were starting to see the truth that abortionists are the real victimizers who operate as if they are above the law.

While Tiller's murder seemed to halt our gains, any setback was only temporary.

During the 2010 midterm elections, those new pro-life Americans took to the polls and voted in an army of newly minted pro-life legislators, who flooded statehouses in 2011 with an unprecedented wave of pro-life bills. Another Gallup poll taken in May 2012 showed that those who identified themselves as "pro-choice" fell to a new low of 41 percent, while pro-life Americans comprised an even half of our citizens.

Then came the trial of Pennsylvania abortionist Kermit Gosnell in 2013. Cheryl attended much of the trial and wrote daily of the gripping, and often grisly, testimony of former clinic workers who described in shocking detail the crimes committed at his squalid West Philadelphia abortion mill. She called on her experience with late-term abortions in Kansas to craft her reports with insight that others lacked. Her stories helped launch a *tweetfest* that shamed the national mainstream media into covering the case.

Soon everyone was talking about abortion abuses, which were covered in graphic detail never before seen on the nightly news. State legislatures, armed with the Gosnell revelations and the understanding that he was not alone, sought new ways to end the barbaric practice of late-term abortion and impose additional regulation on an industry that had run amok for forty years over the lives of women and their babies.

Violence cannot be the answer to humanity's problems, as we see so clearly illustrated in the horror of late-term abortions as much as in the murder of the man who rose to infamy doing them. When the law is taken into the hands of the individual, whether it is an abortionist who thinks he is above the law or a troubled man looking for his fifteen minutes of fame, everyone suffers on both sides of the abortion debate.

Pro-life gains are made when we shine the light of truth on the wickedness of abortion. If you are looking for a formula for ending abortion, look no further than Ephesians 5:11, which tells us to have nothing to do with the unfruitful deeds of darkness, but rather to expose them. Our work in Kansas is the proof that it works.

21

THE NEUHAUS POSTSCRIPT

Let us not become weary in doing good, for at the proper time we will reap a harvest if we do not give up.

—**GALATIANS 6:9**

It had been over a year since Tiller had died and his abortion clinic closed, and we busied ourselves with projects in other states. We were compiling documented evidence against abortionists and learning more about the sordid history of some of the nation's worst. One day, Cheryl curiously received a letter from the Kansas State Board of Healing Arts. Why would the KSBHA be contacting her? We thought all of the complaints from the Tiller era had been closed. We were wrong.

The letter was from Kelli Stevens, the KSBHA litigation counsel who now served as executive director.

> I am writing to inform you of the outcome of investigation which was opened after you filed a complaint regarding Dr. Tiller and Neuhaus. As you are aware, the Board dismissed its disciplinary proceeding against Dr. Tiller after his death. The Board filed a Petition for disci-

> plinary action against Dr. Neuhaus' medical license on April 16, 2010. The matter is currently pending before the Kansas Office of Administrative Hearings. An evidentiary hearing will likely be scheduled in the future. If you have any questions, please feel free to call me.

The news was a legitimate surprise. We were high-fiving and dancing in victory.

Medical boards tend to move at a glacial pace, and the waiting is sometimes the worst part of the process. It took until September 2011 for the disciplinary hearing to actually take place. Cheryl attended every day and reported on the proceedings.

The hearing was conducted in a manner similar to any other court proceeding. Presiding officer Edward Gaschler acted as judge. Reese Hays, a handsome young board litigation attorney with a straightforward, military-like bearing, served as the lead prosecutor. Longtime attorney Robert Eye, a crusty pro-abortion Democrat who had also represented Planned Parenthood, served as Neuhaus's defense attorney. Neuhaus herself appeared at the proceedings frumpy and disheveled—and more than slightly annoyed with the entire affair.

The case revolved around eleven medical records of young women who had received abortions at twenty-five weeks gestation or later. They were the same group of files that had been obtained through a hard-fought subpoena by former attorney general Phill Kline. The women who were the subjects of the abortion records ranged in age from ten to eighteen years of age and were assigned numbers for reference during the proceedings.

Eye started the proceedings by objecting to a KSBHA expert, Dr. Liza H. Gold, who is a respected authority in psychiatry and has contributed to textbooks used to train psychiatrists today. Eye argued that Dr. Gold was unqualified to speak to standard of care issues in Kansas because she does not live in that state and cannot understand the specific nuances of how psychiatry is practiced there. Judge Gaschler rejected this argument since the standard of care does not vary from one geographical location to another.

Next, Eye requested dismissal of ten out of the eleven counts against Neuhaus because the applicable Kansas law, which has since been replaced with more stringent restrictions, referred to risks to a pregnant *woman*. Eye reasoned that since ten out of eleven females were under age eighteen, they did not qualify as women; therefore, abortions done on them were not subject to the law.

Hays appeared to be taken aback by Eye's outlandish argument, but had the presence of mind to note that the definition of a woman would include all females of childbearing age. The judge rejected this outrageous argument of Eye's also.

Eye spent much of the trial attempting to sow general confusion in the court with numerous nonsensical objections, most of which were soon withdrawn.

Without a doubt, Dr. Gold's testimony was devastating to Neuhaus. Gold described an outdated computer program used by Neuhaus, called PsychManager Lite, which had supposedly documented the mental health diagnoses that were used to justify the eleven abortions at issue. This particular D-tree program had never achieved wide popularity because of the issues created by inputting yes or no answers into the program, which would then drop the answers into a psychiatric diagnosis. For example, the computer may ask the question, "Have you experienced weight loss or weight gain in the past six weeks?" If the answer was yes, that would be inputted into the program. However, there was no distinguishing whether the yes answer referred to a weight loss or a gain. Certainly weight gain in the third trimester of pregnancy is a normal, expected occurrence for women, yet the D-tree program counted it as a possible indication of mental illness. This alone made the program completely unreliable.

Today, the program is used only as a teaching tool. Its printouts were never meant to replace the proper medical records of an in-depth mental health evaluation, yet there was no sign in the records that Neuhaus ever did such evaluations.

Dr. Gold also testified that her review of Neuhaus's 2006 inquisition testimony and 2009 trial testimony in the Tiller criminal case only strengthened her opinion that Neuhaus never met the standard of care in the eleven late-term abortion referrals before the board. She further opined that Neuhaus lacked proper training to make such adolescent mental health diagnoses. According to Gold, all the patients should have been referred to a specialist. However, there was no record that Neuhaus had made any referral to anyone for anything.

These were critical points. By law, Tiller needed a referral by a second physician to agree that each post-viability abortion was medically necessary to prevent a "substantial and irreversible impairment to a major bodily function" of the pregnant woman. In each and every case, Neuhaus found no physical risk to the patient, but based her opinion that the abortion was medically necessary on the dubious mental health diagnosis churned out by her PsychManager Lite program.

Mr. Hays questioned Dr. Gold methodically about each file. She described the conditions that the eleven women faced. One fifteen-year-old New York teen sought an abortion in her twenty-eighth week of pregnancy simply because she was "shocked" to learn she was pregnant. Another teen was twenty-six weeks along and wanted an abortion so she could participate in a rodeo as a barrel rider. Another fifteen-year-old loved basketball and sought an abortion because her pregnancy, which had advanced into the third trimester, took the fun out of the sport.

Dr. Paul McHugh, the expert who reviewed the abortion records for attorney general Phill Kline, had earlier been reamed in the media for stating publicly that it was his professional opinion that Tiller performed abortions for "trivial reasons." He had been right all along.

But some of the young ladies faced more serious situations. A ten-year-old girl from California was a rape and incest victim who was twenty-nine weeks pregnant when she was seen by Neuhaus at Tiller's clinic. Another was a fifteen-year-old teen in her twenty-sixth week of pregnancy who made conflicting statements concerning suicidal thoughts. An eighteen-year-old Kansas woman who was twenty-five weeks along had a history of panic attacks. Neuhaus labeled her "unable to function" even though the record stated she regularly attended school and work.

Dr. Gold stated that it was her professional opinion that Neuhaus violated the standard of care in each of the eleven late-term abortion cases, noting that Neuhaus should have referred all eleven patients to either experts in child psychology or specialists in adolescent psychology.

Cross-examination of Dr. Gold really didn't help Neuhaus's cause. Eye questioned Dr. Gold about standard of care for mental health evaluations for late-term abortions. Dr. Gold replied that there is no such thing. "Late-term abortion is not a treatment or intervention for any psychiatric condition," she explained.

When questioned about whether she had ever admitted a patient to the hospital for a late-term abortion, Dr. Gold responded, "It would be inappropriate for a psychiatrist to admit a patient to a hospital for abortion services."

Eye then explored whether an unwanted pregnancy put a teen at risk for developing psychiatric disorders. Again, Dr. Gold's answer was emphatic. "Teen pregnancy is not a risk factor for psychiatric disorders," she said.

It became clear that Tiller and Neuhaus had created phony mental health excuses based on shoddy or nonexistent mental health evaluations to justify third-trimester abortions that would have otherwise been illegal in Kansas. In fact, since none of the women met the requirement of facing a substantial and irreversible condition—physical or mental—

the late-term abortions done at Tiller's clinic were blatantly illegal, and, given Tiller's careful control and oversight of his abortion business, it appeared there was no way he could not have known that.

This also meant that Phill Kline's original thirty criminal charges of illegal late-term abortion filed against Tiller, only to be dropped by district attorney Nola Foulston the next day, were validated and would have very likely led to a criminal conviction, had Tiller been tried on those counts.

After the prosecution's case, it was time for Robert Eye to go to work. He called Neuhaus to the stand.

We heard her testimony. It took only about five minutes of listening to her speak to understand that she was not what one would expect or desire from a licensed physician. Her appearance was shabby and unkempt—and maybe even a little bit dirty. She often rambled off topic and would sometimes mutter to herself in Gollum-like fashion instead of directly answering questions. Her public behavior was shockingly unprofessional, alternating between the persona of a wounded animal and a venomous snake about to strike, hissing paranoid accusations and indignant defenses. I found it frightening that she was ever involved in providing any kind of medical care to patients.

Neuhaus gave often rambling and unfocused testimony to defend the lack of information contained in her medical files about the patients in question. Several patients with widely varying circumstances had identical computer printouts in their records as the only evidence of Neuhaus's interaction with them. One file lacked any diagnosis, and another file indicated the diagnosis was generated days after the abortion, raising questions that both abortions were illegally done.

Neuhaus blamed her omission of critical record contents required by Kansas Administrative Regulations on pro-life activists. She feared that one day the records might fall into the hands of Attorney General Phill Kline or other pro-lifers.

It was nothing more than a "boogeyman" defense. No patient identities were ever made public. The records were subjected to more security precautions than the nation's nuclear secrets. Nobody really cared who those patients were. That was beside the point. It was just a tactic to use the fear of privacy breaches to excuse Neuhaus's shoddy medical practices.

Her attitude that she was above the law exposed the thinking that is indicative of today's abortion cartel. "I'm here to comply with the law, but once I step into the clinic, my own priorities take precedence," she stated.

Today's headlines are replete with abortion clinics, such as those in Mississippi, Alabama, Pennsylvania, and Virginia, that resist regulation and oversight while demanding that they should not have to comply with standards with which other medical facilities must comply. This unwillingness to respect and abide by the law makes abortion clinics dangerous places for women because it strips away their protections, which state laws attempt to provide.

In the end, it became obvious that Neuhaus's mental health determinations were a sham and little more than a "rubber stamp" for Tiller so he could continue providing abortions through the latest term of pregnancy. The presiding officer agreed.

Gaschler issued his initial order in February 2012, recommending the revocation of Neuhaus's Kansas medical license and ordering her to pay for the costs of the proceedings, which came close to one hundred thousand dollars. Gaschler noted that Neuhaus's shoddy record keeping and her inadequate mental health evaluations of the pregnant women fell well below the standards of care. "The care and treatment of the 11 patients in question was seriously jeopardized by the Licensee's care," he wrote (John Hanna, "Loss of license ordered in Kansas abortion-referrals case," NBCNews.com, February 21, 2012, http://www.nbcnews.com/id/46474681/ns/health/t/loss-license

-ordered-kansas-abortion-referrals-case/#.UxX4nz9dWSo).

Judge Gaschler's order was finalized with a unanimous vote of the board in June 2012. I was flooded with emotions as I sat in the gallery and listened to the vote, because I understood that the revocation of Neuhaus's license was also an indictment of guilt against Tiller.

I had uprooted my family, leaving our beloved California home to assail the enemy in his stronghold in an effort the likes of which had never been done on this scale. I endured the painful wounds of "friendly fire" and sometimes brutal attacks from the enemy. But we overcame every hurdle, including government corruption and a negative press. We helped give the pro-life movement a new sense that victory was possible.

Our Wichita project, which I thought would take a year—maybe two—consumed nearly a decade. It was some of the most difficult and challenging work of my life, but that day, sitting before the Kansas Board of Healing Arts, I felt that I'd finally won.

PART 3

NUTS AND BOLTS

22

JUST THE FACTS

I am a firm believer in the people. If given the truth, they can be depended upon to meet any national crisis. The great point is to bring them the real facts.

—**ABRAHAM LINCOLN**

When we first arrived in Wichita, we tried to learn everything we could about the abortion clinics in that community. In doing so, we ran across what we call "pro-life folklore."

Pro-life folklore is a story handed down by word of mouth over the years about the history of abortion in a particular community. While it is likely the story has been embellished or altered in the telling, it is considered gospel nonetheless. There were many stories that began like this: "My sister-in-law's cousin was at the hair salon and heard from the lady in the next chair that . . ."

You get the picture. The stories seemed to take on lives of their own.

Cheryl's job was to research the abortion clinics and debunk the folklore. We had a rule that if we did not have a piece of paper to back it up, the story—no matter how salacious—did not get repeated and it did not get published. Eventually, her research turned into a seventy-two-page booklet summarizing documentable facts about the local abortion mills. It became a "go-to" resource for pro-lifers, who used it for sidewalk counseling, in writing to legislators and newspaper editors, for public speaking, when giving interviews, or even in just discussing abortion with friends and family.

There is a common perception in the pro-abortion liberal crowd that pro-life activists are uneducated, religiously bigoted, woman-hating knuckle-draggers who have no tether on reality or the truth about abortion. Too often, our side gives them fodder for continuing that belief by spouting "facts" that are really folklore.

Even the most well-meaning people fall into this trap. Recently Republican senator Jon Kyl of Arizona, a pro-life stalwart, received a firestorm of criticism when he stated that abortion is "well over 90 percent of what Planned Parenthood does." While pro-life supporters understand that Planned Parenthood is the largest provider of abortions in the United States, the 90 percent figure was immediately shot down as false, and it gave Planned Parenthood a golden media opportunity to bash those in the Senate who attempted to defund the organization. Kyl was forced to "walk back" his comments. (See Jason Linkins, "Jon Kyl Is Sorry If He Gave Anyone the Impression that the Things He Says in Public Are Factual," *Huffington Post*, http://www.huffingtonpost.com/2011/04/08/jon-kyl-is-sorry-if-he-ga_n_846941.html.) It was an embarrassing setback.

In this work, credibility is a virtue. People need to trust that what you say is true and that you can back it up. Pro-life activists are held to a high standard, and there are always those who are looking to discredit information from pro-life sources. That is why research and documentation are such an important foundation to your efforts to stop abortion and save lives.

Start with researching the laws in your state. The only way you will know if an abortionist is breaking the law is to first know what the law says.

Don't limit your research to state abortion laws. There are less obvious laws that are just as applicable to abortion clinics. Look up health code regulations that that may pertain to medical offices. Learn the legal requirements for medical waste removal and human tissue disposal. Check on zoning requirements for the abortion clinic neighborhoods. There are regulations businesses must follow for handicap access, adequate parking spaces, or even proper signage.

Make sure you don't waste your precious research time by relying solely on your memory. No one wants to do a job twice!

Keep files of your findings on your computer or hard copies in a binder or file cabinet for easy reference. Highlight the relevant statutes or ordinances that you think might be useful. Use sticky notes and colorful tabs to help you more easily find relevant portions of the law. This record will become a prized resource as you learn more about abortion practices in your area and how the law applies to them.

Once you have a basic understanding of abortion laws in your state, find out which regulatory agency is responsible for enforcement. Every state is a little different, so learning which agencies are responsible for various aspects of an abortion operation is critical in getting the laws enforced.

As a general rule of thumb, medical boards are responsible for physician oversight. Health departments are generally responsible for the actions and condition of the abortion facility.

When we began our work in Wichita, we were shocked to learn that there was absolutely no oversight mechanism in place for holding abortion facilities accountable for maintaining health and safety standards. Because of this, Krishna Rajanna was able to operate an appallingly filthy abortion mill in Kansas City where procedure rooms featured bloodstained carpeting. His clinic was so dirty that one police detective who visited the clinic would not sit down on the grimy waiting room chairs.

But Rajanna's squalor was not unique, by any means.

After we bought the Central Women's Services building in Wichita and closed that business in 2006, we learned that no inspector had ever darkened the doorway of that run-down abortion mill in the twenty-three years it had operated in that location. Conditions there were so unsanitary that we had to completely strip the interior down to the rafters and cinder block, sandblast the walls and ceiling, then completely rebuild it from the ground up in order to be able to use it as our new headquarters.

We aggressively exposed these abortion abuses and lobbied for abortion clinic accountability. Because we understood the deficiencies in the law, we were able to do something about it. As a result, the Kansas Legislature passed a clinic licensing law in 2011 that has put responsibility for abortion clinic oversight under the authority of the Kansas Department of Health and Environment, which now has the authority to close abortion clinics that do not comply with the state's tough new abortion clinic safety standards.

WHAT YOU WILL NEED TO GET STARTED:

- a computer
- an Internet connection
- a printer
- ability to use a search engine
- time to invest in research
- a file box or cabinet to store your documentation for easy access

23

IDENTIFY AND RESEARCH YOUR LOCAL ABORTIONIST

Know your enemy and know yourself and you can fight a hundred battles without disaster.

—**SUN TZU**

It is very common for us to hear from the dear pro-life warrior who has been standing outside his local abortion clinic for years, but has no idea who is actually working inside. Not every clinic has a famous abortionist like James Scott Pendergraft in Florida, or Martin Haskell in Ohio. Some abortion businesses work very hard to conceal their abortionists' identities. Sometimes there is such a turnover in staffing that it is hard to keep up with the frequent personnel changes.

We have painstakingly done much of that research for you.

A few years ago, as we intensified our work in several states, we discovered that no one had a realistic idea how many abortion clinics were left in this country. There was even less knowledge about who staffed them. Most of the lists were out of date or just not complete. We conducted a research project over three years aimed at listing every abortion clinic in the nation. We expanded the project to eventually include abortionists and where they worked.

In the process, we began to amass a huge amount of data on the abortion cartel. We discovered that in 1991 there were 2,176 abortion clinics in America. Since then more than 70 percent of all surgical abortion clinics have closed for good. That represented a stunning victory for the pro-life movement of which most were completely unaware. In fact, the prevailing thought was that the pro-life movement had more failures than successes. Our research proved the opposite. The work to stop abortion has made significant headway and actually has the abortion cartel on the ropes. The volumes of documents detailing abortion abuses and disciplinary action that we were acquiring proved it.

Our challenge was to develop a platform to get the information we'd acquired through years of careful research into the hands of other pro-life organizations, activists, and the public.

Thus, AbortionDocs.org was born. This website is a searchable database of every surgical abortion clinic, every medication abortion clinic, and every known abortionist in the nation. But it is more than a list. Each entry has a profile page that includes photos and links to documents—to the extent that they are available—that prove involvement in abortion abuses and other outlandish behavior. We continue to gather information and update the site daily. It is an amazing resource for the pro-life movement, which can now quantify successes instead of focusing on failures.

The website also keeps a running total of the number of abortion clinics and known abortionists. From these statistics, we can actually watch the number of abortion clinics drop from day to day. This is an incredibly encouraging feature for our friends, and it is equally demoralizing to the enemies of life.

When researching your local abortion clinic, one of the first places you should search is AbortionDocs.org. This could save you valuable time since every document we have has been made available online. Items may include photos of the abortion clinic, photos of medical emergency incidents, videos produced by activists and news stations, audio recordings of 911 calls, medical license applications, abortionists' disciplinary action forms, health department deficiency reports, lawsuit documents, and links to published articles.

While every abortion clinic in the country can be found at AbortionDocs.org, not every abortionist is listed. This is because of frequent changes in abortion clinic staffing and the industry's proclivity for concealing their abortionists' identities. If a particular abortionist is not listed on AbortionDocs.org, you will just have to dig a little deeper.

The first place you should search is the medical board site in your state. A handy URL that will help you conduct a license lookup is www.docboard.org/docfinder.html. This site has links to every medical board site in the nation. You can find all kinds of useful information there. If an abortionist has been disciplined, it will be noted on his or her profile page. Download the disciplinary documents for future reference. (We will discuss this in detail later.)

Next, try a Google search of the clinic and abortionist by name to see what turns up. Search social networking sites such as Facebook, Twitter, and LinkedIn. Sometimes very interesting insight can be garnered from their social network profiles, including photos of the abortionists doing crazy things. For example, the administrator of an abortion chain in Texas left her social profile public, and we found a ridiculous photo of the bleached blonde—dark roots embarrassingly showing—making a silly face while peering through a curtain of plastic grass. That picture made her look like anything but the serious medical professional she purported herself to be. We have used the photo repeatedly on our own website.

Look for lawsuits, criminal records, and mentions in old news stories. These often show up on Google searches but can also be found in the court records at your local courthouse. You never know what you might find. We have discovered mundane records, such as speeding tickets, divorce records, and tax records, but we have also discovered significant information, such as restraining orders, evidence of spousal abuse, and sometimes even criminal history and nonpayment of taxes on a home and/or business.

Study your local abortion clinic's website to familiarize yourself with exactly how it is marketing abortions to women. Find out how late in pregnancy they do abortions, what procedures they use, and other such information you may find useful.

Make sure you check their online informed consent forms, if they have them. Some states require the names of the abortionists to be listed on them.

Following is a sample abortion consent form as it appears for an actual Kansas abortion business. We have changed the name and contact information; however, all of the misspellings, errors, and snide comments concerning several aspects of the information they are required to share with potential abortion clients are original to the actual document, and are themselves a commentary on the shoddy nature of the abortion cartel.

Try searching for your abortion clinic by name on the secretary of state's website in your state. Most of them have a searchable database that includes information about the owner and officers involved in every business in the state and the status of the business's license. However, if your local abortionist is an independent contractor, he or she would probably not show up in those records—although other information there could prove useful.

SAMPLE ABORTION CONSENT FORM

ABC Abortion Clinic, 24-Hour Form
123 Main St., Kansas City, KS 66100, [phone number]

BRING THIS FORM WITH YOU to your appointment at ABC Abortion Clinic.

Re-printing this form the night before appointment will change timestamp and make this form worthless.

The "Women's Right To Know" Act of July 1st, 1997 (now K.S.A. 65-6709): Voluntary and informed consent for an elective abortion is required unless it can be shown that you need a therapeutic abortion to save your life because of a medical emergency. For "voluntary and informed consent" we must provide you in writing at least 24 hours prior to your abortion:

1. DOCTOR'S NAME (KSA 65-6709(a)(1)) – John Doe, MD.

2. PROCEDURE DESCRIPTION (KSA 65-6709(a)(2)) – The most common kind of abortion we do is by suction aspiration. After injecting a local anesthetic around the cervix, a series of tapered dilator rods, each a little wider than the one before, are inserted and removed to stretch the cervix open wider and then insert a cannula tube into the uterus. Suction is then applied to the cannula tube while gently removing the pregnancy tissue from the uterus. We may use a tear-drop shaped curette to dislodge any tissue that may still remain. The uterus is then re-suctioned to remove any remaining tissue. If you do not dilate easily (at 11 weeks LMP or more) we will insert misoprostol tablets between your cheek and gums and have you wait 2–3 hours for cervical dilation. Later, we will do a regular suction aspiration abortion as described.

3. POSSIBLE COMPLICATIONS (KSA 65-6709(a)(3)) – a.) Infections, which are usually avoided if the woman observes her follow-up instructions and takes her preventative antibiotics; b.) Unlikely tear in the cervix, which may be repaired with stitches. That may cause an increased risk of premature delivery in the future; c.) Anesthesia or other medication allergic reactions; d.) Perforation of the uterine wall and possibly other organs (less than 0.1%), which may heal themselves or may require surgical repair; e.) An incomplete abortion (approximately 1–2%) or in which blood clots accumulate in the uterus (1%) requiring removal; and finally, f.) Excessive bleeding (less than 0.1%) which may require a blood transfusion. Serious complications are rare. First trimester abortions are safer than carrying to full-term. The mortality rate with legal abortions is 0.91 per 100,000 abortions. Homicide of pregnant and post-partum females by their male partners is 1.7 per 100,000. Risks to future reproductive health from an abortion are associated with a chlamydia or gonorrhea infection severe enough to cause Fallopian tube scarring (acquired prior to the abortion), or a perforation of the uterus and the resulting hysterectomy that might have to be done (highly unlikely).

14. NO PAYMENT REQUIRED BEFORE 24th HOUR (KSA 65-6709(g)) – by law we cannot require you to pay for the abortion during the 24 hours after receiving this information, but this does not stop us from requiring payment after the 24th hour and before the abortion.

By signing below, you acknowledge that you have read and understood the information above, and that you received this information at least 24-hours prior to your abortion (KSA 65-6709(d-e)).

______________________________ Signed and received

Manta.com is another great site for looking up an abortion business, although sometimes the information can be somewhat outdated. Usually you will be able to find out who the clinic's registered agent is, how many employees it has, and the general yearly income of the business.

Be creative in your searches. Search in various ways. On local news sites, search the clinic's and abortionist's name, but also search more generic terms, such as "abortion" or "women's health" to see what turns up. If your local abortionist works in more than one state, check out news sites, business listings, and license information in each state and community.

Make a file on your hard drive and a paper file to keep the results of your searches. Something that may seem insignificant right now may have greater implications later. Sometimes it is nearly impossible to relocate old information that is needed if a significant amount of time has passed. You will never regret taking the time to archive your research.

If your Internet research doesn't yield the information you are looking for, don't get discouraged. There are other options.

RESEARCH TIPS:

- Bookmark and use AbortionDocs.org.
- Bookmark and use http://www.docboard.org/docfinder.html for physician license information.
- Become familiar with your local clinic's website and consent forms.
- Search social networking sites for your local clinic and provider.
- Check the secretary of state's online business search for business status and other important information related to your local abortion clinic.
- Be creative in your searches, and use many different keywords to refine your searches.
- Create a file on your computer's hard drive where you can save the results of your research so you don't have to do it over.
- Print important documentation, web pages, or other information, and keep a hard copy in a file box or cabinet for easy reference.

24

THE UNDERCOVER CALL

"All warfare is based on deception." —**SUN TZU**

One of the easiest ways to get the information you need is through the "undercover call." It takes a little forethought, but it can be incredibly fruitful.

How is it done? During the call, you pretend to be a pregnant woman who wants an abortion. If you are a man, or perhaps a bit too mature to pull that scenario off, you can pretend you are a pregnant teen's dad or mom, calling on her behalf with questions.

Some activists are more squeamish than others about making up stories for these calls. Some have no problem whatsoever stretching the truth to a godless enemy who is bent on destroying innocent lives—especially if it can be used to save babies. One need only look at the story of Rahab in the Bible for an example of a woman who used misdirection to save the lives of the Jewish spies and was honored by God for it (See Joshua 2).

However, others have moral compunctions against such things. We are not asking anyone to violate his or her conscience. The undercover call is a tool that you can choose to use or not. If you do decide it is for you, we have some helpful tips.

First, get a notepad and jot down the name you want to use for the woman seeking an abortion. Determine her age and figure out an appropriate date of birth. Then decide if this is a first-, second-, or third-trimester abortion you are seeking. The later the gestation, the more detailed your backstory needs to be in order to sound credible. Use a pregnancy calculator from the Internet (use Google to find one), and backtrack to arrive at a date for the last menstrual period (LMP). You should also have a fictitious address, including zip code, and a telephone number.

If it is legal to do so in your state, we highly recommend that you record the call. There is no telling what kind of information a chatty receptionist might drop. Sometimes these calls actually catch clinic workers doing illegal things. In that case, your recording could be used as evidence and turned over to the proper authorities. There are some handy digital audio recorders on the market that have USB capabilities. They allow you to plug your recorder directly into your computer, where you can permanently save the audio files of your conversations. Some smartphones and computers have built-in audio recorders. If you use an iPhone, its voice recorder will allow you to text and e-mail audio files—which can be handy. However, to use that app, you will have to place the call from another phone.

We also recommend that you block the call by pressing *67 on your telephone keypad before dialing the number. In this age of caller ID, that can protect your privacy. But heed a word of warning.

Once, I placed a call to an abortion clinic from a toll-free 800 line in our office. I blocked the call, or so I thought, using *67. I then engaged in a big conversation with a clinic worker, who eventually asked me to identify myself. I made up a name and said I was a reporter.

"That's funny," said the receptionist. "My caller ID says this is Operation Rescue."

Now flummoxed, I replied, "Well, that's strange. I don't know why it would say that." Then I hung up as if the handset had suddenly become a hot potato. We laughed so hard about that, but we learned a new thing. Calls from 800 numbers cannot be blocked using the *67 code.

When you are ready, make the call and schedule an abortion. Before the conversation ends, ask who you or your daughter will be seeing. Sometimes this works like a charm.

A few years ago, our assistant called a particularly seedy abortion clinic in Los Angeles, scheduled an appointment, and then asked who she would be seeing. The receptionist told her that "Dr. Steve" would be doing her abortion. "Dr. Steve" turned out to be an unlicensed clinic worker who was performing abortions at several clinics in Southern California. We filed a complaint with the California medical board. When we followed up a few weeks later, we discovered that "Dr. Steve" was no longer employed by the abortion clinic chain and had disappeared. We have searched for him frequently over the years, but the man just dropped off the radar, most likely out of fear of criminal charges for impersonating a doctor and performing illegal abortions.

Once Cheryl walked into a new clinic in Chula Vista, California, and picked up their business card. It listed four abortionists. After a little research, we found out that all of the abortionists had troubled pasts. One of them was a convicted sex offender who was caught molesting his abortion patients while they were vulnerable. Our research gave us the documentation we needed to expose the ugly truth about this abortion clinic to the community. All four of the abortionists listed on that card eventually lost their medical licenses due to public pressure brought by pro-life supporters and the negative press we generated for them.

We have also discovered the identities of abortionists through a variety of other means, such as talking to patients or clinic workers. Just keep trying and do not give up. Eventually you will find what you need.

Sometimes you have to put the puzzle pieces together. During our efforts in Wichita, we learned that Tiller had hired a new abortionist. He printed monthly calendars on his website with the last names of his abortion staff printed on each day they worked. This was to satisfy a legal requirement that a patient had to be informed who would do her abortion at least twenty-four hours in advance.

The new abortionist was listed simply as Robinson. One local group jumped to the erroneous conclusion that Tiller had hired Texas abortionist Lamar Robinson, and began to spread that assumption around. We were less convinced. Lamar Robinson is a black man, and we never saw anyone matching his description at the clinic. Besides, there was no record that he was licensed in Kansas. We prayed for an answer to this riddle.

One day soon after, we got a call from a sidewalk counselor. A woman had tossed torn-up pieces of paper out her window before driving away from the abortion clinic. The sidewalk counselor had retrieved them and gave them to us. We pieced them together and discovered the initials *S. R.* on a line that required a physician's signature. We went to the "Search for a Licensee" option on the Kansas State Board of Healing Arts website and searched the name "Robinson." Up popped an entry for Susan C. Robinson—the only S. Robinson in the database at the time. A quick Google search showed she was a Planned Parenthood circuit-riding abortionist from California. Our prayers were answered and the puzzle was solved!

As the Spanish say, "Quién busca, halla"—whoever seeks, finds.

WHEN MAKING AN UNDERCOVER CALL:

- Make sure recording phone conversations is legal in your state.
- Acquire a digital audio recorder with USB capability.
- Make notes on your "backstory," including your name, age, date of birth, date of last menstrual cycle, and so forth.
- Make a list of questions you would like to have answered.
- Learn how to block your phone number, and make sure to do it.
- Ask for the name of the provider you would be seeing during your "appointment."
- Take notes during the conversation of any important points as a memory aid.
- Maintain a copy of the audio file on your computer for your records.

25

LICENSE LOOKUP

Ask and it will be given to you; seek and you will find; knock and the door will be opened to you.

—**LUKE 11:9**

Once you find out who your local abortionist is, you can look him or her up on your state's medical board licensing website. Usually there will be a button that says something like "Look for a Licensee" where you can begin your search. (As previously mentioned, www.docboard.org/docfinder.html has links to medical boards in every state. Bookmark it for future reference.)

When you locate the practitioner on the website, you will find information about the status of his or her medical license, as well as whether there has been any discipline, typically in the past ten years. Most states will have links to the actual disciplinary documents, which are usually filled with all kinds of useful information.

If your state does not keep disciplinary documents online, there will be instructions on the website telling you how to get them. Just follow the directions.

Every physician that is licensed must file an application for licensure. The applications contain information about the physician's educational and employment histories, hospital affiliations, disciplinary histories, and some limited information about malpractice claims. Every couple of years, licensees must fill out a renewal application where they must update the board on their current address, criminal convictions, and any large malpractice claims they have incurred since their last renewal. These applications are public records that can be obtained by writing a simple letter of request to the appropriate state's medical board.

In 2010, news broke that New Jersey abortionist Steven Chase Brigham was operating a secret illegal late-term abortion clinic in Elkton, Maryland. Authorities discovered it when one of Brigham's associates, Nicola Irene Riley, botched an abortion so badly that the patient was transported by Life Flight to a hospital in Baltimore, where she underwent emergency surgery to save her life. Riley had punctured her womb, pulled a bowel, and shoved parts of the dismembered baby into the woman's abdominal cavity. We immediately ordered Riley's medical license application from Maryland.

Our assistant came in one day and told us that the application had arrived. We asked if it said anything interesting. "Oh, just something about a criminal conviction and time in jail," she casually replied. Our jaws dropped and it was a race to see who could grab the documents first.

We immediately began to publish a series of articles exposing Riley's background. I made an open records request to the United States Army for her military criminal records.

Through these records, we discovered that Riley had told medical boards in Maryland, Wyoming, and her home state of Utah that while serving in the military, she had failed to report in a timely manner a credit card/identity theft ring that was being run by soldiers under her command. For that she said she was convicted of conduct unbecoming an officer and served one year in a federal military prison.

Once we got the records from the Army, we discovered that Riley had actually been the ringleader and main perpetrator. She would obtain personal information of other soldiers during her military duties, then use that information to apply for credit cards, with which she bought large amounts of expensive jewelry and other items. She actually served three years, not one, at the Fort Leavenworth military prison in Kansas.

We reported this discrepancy to the medical boards in all three states where Riley held active medical licenses, as well as in Virginia, where she had a pending license application. As a result, Maryland, which had already suspended Riley's license after that horrifically botched abortion in Elkton, added additional charges of lying to the board in order to gain licensure. Wyoming ordered Riley to surrender her license or face revocation proceedings. Utah banned her from doing abortions, and Virginia denied her application for a license in that state.

You never know what nugget of information you will get from a license application or where it will lead next. These applications are well worth the trouble of asking for them. Operation Rescue has already obtained many abortionists' license applications, and they are available for viewing and download at AbortionDocs.org.

Make it a habit to regularly check on the status of your local abortionists on the license lookup link in your state. By doing this, you will be among the first to know if any disciplinary action has been taken and when the disciplinary hearings might be. These hearings are usually open to the public.

If possible, make every effort to attend disciplinary hearings for abortionists in your area. Sometimes the hearings are conducted like trials, complete with a hearing officer (who acts as the judge), prosecutors, defense attorneys, and witness testimony.

It is the witness testimony that can be extremely valuable. For example, a disciplinary hearing was held for late-term abortionist Shelley Sella, who was charged with gross neglect in a case involving a life-threatening complication on a patient who was thirty-five weeks pregnant. Sella was accused of ignoring medical history that included a previous Cesarean-section delivery, which made inducing labor a high-risk procedure that should not have been done at an outpatient facility. Sella proceeded with the abortion anyway. The woman suffered a ruptured uterus and was rushed to the hospital, where another physician conducted emergency surgery that saved her life.

The disciplinary charges came as the result of complaints filed by Cheryl and by Tara Shaver of Project Defending Life, who obtained 911 calls through Freedom of Information requests that revealed the botched abortion.

The New Mexico Medical Board closed the hearing but later released full transcripts of the proceedings, which were very useful in better understanding the abortion method, use of dangerous drugs such as Cytotec (an ulcer drug used off-label by abortionists to "ripen" the cervix and induce labor), and general abortion protocols.

The expert witness for the prosecution had volumes to say about the dangers of Sella's outpatient third-trimester abortion practices. While Sella was mysteriously cleared of all wrongdoing in the botched abortion, the information garnered from the hearing has been of great use to the pro-life movement.

This kind of information can not only help save lives locally, but can aid the pro-life movement as a whole to better understand current abortion protocols and procedures. This can lead to legislation and greater oversight and, in some cases, banning of certain practices, as was done with the partial-birth abortion procedure. Federal law passed in 2004 brought a halt to this grisly abortion method after pro-life research brought it to the public's attention.

USING A LICENSE LOOKUP SITE:

- Make sure you spell the provider's name correctly.
- If unsure of the proper spelling, try variations until you get it right.
- Save any disciplinary documents available online to your hard drive for easy future reference.
- If disciplinary documents are not available online, make a FOIA request for them using information provided online.
- Request copies of transcripts of any disciplinary hearings.
- Request copies of license applications.
- If lawsuits or criminal convictions are listed, do further research on them.
- If you confirm that an abortion provider is unlicensed or operating under a suspended license, immediately file a formal complaint along with your documentation to the medical board.

26

THE ELECTRONIC SLEUTH

Information is the oxygen of the modern age. It seeps through the walls topped by barbed wire, it wafts across the electrified borders.

—**RONALD REAGAN**

It is amazing what can be found on the Internet these days. What is better is that the information is free for the taking.

If you don't already know how, learn how to use a search engine, such as Google or Yahoo. You can usually discover some pretty astonishing things about your local abortion business in just a few minutes of searching.

For example, let's say you are using the Google search engine. In the box on the main page, type in a keyword, such as "Kentucky abortion complications," or the name of the abortion clinic in your hometown. If nothing useful comes up in the list generated by your search, try refining your search or using other keywords. If you use too general a keyword, such as "abortion," you might scroll through dozens of pages of results and never find what you are looking for, so try to keep your searches as specific as possible.

Most state medical boards publish disciplinary documents online, which can be downloaded at no cost. The same goes for abortion clinic deficiency reports prepared by health departments. Most of the documents available through government agencies, with a few exceptions, are public record; therefore you have a right to them. If there is something you need from an agency that cannot be found online, just call or e-mail them and ask for it.

Another great thing to search for is public statements by abortionists. When abortionists talk, they usually say ridiculous things. Document their interviews and writings; then learn to use their own words against them. Search for interviews and articles that quote, or are written by, your local abortionist or clinic staffer. Keep a file of these for future reference. These quotes can be used in sidewalk counseling brochures, letters to editors and legislators, articles, interviews, speeches, etc., to expose the truth about abortion and those who offer it.

We have employed the tactic of using abortionists' own words against them over and over, with good results. For example, in 2011, Kansas finally passed a clinic licensing law that pro-life groups, including Operation Rescue, had attempted to pass since 2004. During legislative testimony, Overland Park abortionist Herbert Hodes stated that he believed that five women had died from abortions in Kansas in the past five years. The statement was reported by the Associated Press.

We quickly confirmed that only one abortion-related death had been officially reported in the past ten years in Kansas, which led us to believe that Hodes knew something the rest of us didn't. Were abortion deaths going unreported in violation of the law? We demanded investigations.

That put Hodes on the hot seat. He was forced to issue a letter backtracking on his statements, which impugned the veracity of his other statements to the legislature. Despite his efforts to dial back his statements, the damage was done. The safety of women at abortion clinics was called into question. The clinic-licensing bill passed handily and was signed into law.

In another example, one Kansas group took transcripts from LeRoy Carhart's court testimony in defense of the heinous partial-birth abortion, titled it "Carhart Speaks," and turned it into a handout that was given to abortion patients when he worked in Wichita at George Tiller's late-term abortion mill. The testimony was chilling.

ATTORNEY: Are there times when you don't remove the fetus intact?

CARHART: Yes, sir.

ATTORNEY: Can you tell me about that, when that occurs?

CARHART: That occurs when the tissue fragments, or frequently when you rupture the membranes, an arm will spontaneously prolapse through the os. I think most . . . statistically the most common presentation, we talk about the forehead or the skull being first. We talked about the feet being first, but I think in probably the great majority of terminations, it's what they would call a transverse lie, so really you're looking at a side profile of a curved fetus. When the patient . . . the uterus is already starting to contract and they are starting to miscarry, when you rupture the waters, usually something prolapses through the uterine, through the cervical os, not always, but very often an extremity will.

ATTORNEY: What do you do then?

CARHART: My normal course would be to dismember that extremity and then go back and try to take the fetus out either foot or skull first, whatever end I can get to first.

ATTORNEY: How do you go about dismembering that extremity?

CARHART: Just traction and rotation, grasping the portion that you can get a hold of which would be usually somewhere up the shaft of the exposed portion of the fetus, pulling down on it through the os, using the internal os as your counter-traction and rotating to dismember the shoulder or the hip or whatever it would be. Sometimes you will get one leg and you can't get the other leg out.

ATTORNEY: In that situation, are you, when you pull on the arm and remove it, is the fetus still alive?

CARHART: Yes.

ATTORNEY: Do you consider an arm, for example, to be a substantial portion of the fetus?

CARHART: In the way I read it, I think if I lost my arm, that would be a substantial loss to me. I think I would have to interpret it that way.

ATTORNEY: And then what happens next after you remove the arm? You then try to remove the rest of the fetus?

CARHART: Then I would go back and attempt to either bring the feet down or bring the skull down, or even sometimes you bring the other arm down and remove that also and then get the feet down.

ATTORNEY: At what point is the fetus ... does the fetus die during that process?

CARHART: I don't really know. I know that the fetus is alive during the process most of the time because I can see fetal heartbeat on the ultrasound.

THE COURT: Counsel, for what it's worth, it still is unclear to me with regard to the intact D&E when fetal demise occurs.

ATTORNEY: Okay, I will try to clarify that. In the procedure of an intact D&E where you would start foot first, with the situation where the fetus is presented feet first, tell me how you are able to get the feet out first.

CARHART: Under ultrasound, you can see the extremities. You know what is what. You know what the foot is, you know what the arm is, you know what the skull is. By grabbing the feet and pulling down on it or by grabbing a knee and pulling down on it, usually you can get one leg out, get the other leg out and bring the fetus out. I don't know where this . . . all the controversy about rotating the fetus comes from. I don't attempt to do that. I just attempt to bring out whatever is the proximal portion of the fetus.

ATTORNEY: At the time that you bring out the feet in this example, is the fetus still alive?

CARHART: Yes.

ATTORNEY: Then what's the next step you do?

CARHART: I didn't mention it. I should. I usually attempt to grasp the cord first and divide the cord, if I can do that.

ATTORNEY: What is the cord?

CARHART: The cord is the structure that transports the blood, both arterial and venous, from the fetus, and back to the fetus, and it gives the fetus its only source of oxygen, so that if you can divide the cord, the fetus will eventually die, but whether this takes five minutes or fifteen minutes and when that occurs, I don't think anyone really knows.

ATTORNEY: Are there situations where you don't divide the cord?

CARHART: There are situations when I can't.

ATTORNEY: What are those?

CARHART: I just can't get to the cord. It's either high above the fetus and structures where you can't reach up that far. The instruments are only 11 inches long.

ATTORNEY: Let's take the situation where you haven't divided the cord because you couldn't, and you have begun to remove a living fetus feet first. What happens next after you have gotten the feet removed?

CARHART: We remove the feet and continue with traction on the feet until the abdomen and the thorax came through the cavity. At that point, I would try . . . you have to bring the shoulders down, but if you can get enough of them outside, you can do this with your finger outside of the uterus, and then at that point the fetal . . . the base of the fetal skull is usually in the cervical canal.

ATTORNEY: What do you do next?

CARHART: And you can reach that, and that's where you would rupture the fetal skull to some extent and aspirate the contents out.

ATTORNEY: At what point in that process does fetal demise occur between initial remove . . . removal of the feet or legs and the crushing of the skull, or I'm sorry, the decompressing of the skull?

CARHART: Well, you know, again, this is where I'm not sure what fetal demise is. I mean, I honestly have to share your concern, your Honor. You can remove the cranial contents and the fetus will still have a heartbeat for several seconds or several minutes, so is the fetus alive? I would have to say probably, although I don't think it has any brain function, so it's brain dead at that point.

ATTORNEY: So the brain death might occur when you begin suctioning out of the cranium?

CARHART: I think brain death would occur because the suctioning to remove contents is only two or three seconds, so somewhere in that period of time, obviously not when you penetrate the skull, because people get shot in the head and they don't die immediately from that, if they are going to die at all, so that probably is not sufficient to kill the fetus, but I think removing the brain contents eventually will.

("Court testimony on fetal brain harvesting," transcript of July 1997 testimony of LeRoy Carhart, The Tribune Papers, http://www.ashevilletribune.com/archives/tissue/Harvesting.htm)

Later, under cross-examination from the attorney general's counsel, Carhart stated, "My intent in every abortion I have ever done is to kill the fetus and terminate the pregnancy."

It's hard to imagine a person who would not be repulsed by that horrific testimony. Carhart's own words—given under oath and on the records—exposed the heinous act of late-term abortion with such power. Volumes written by pro-life activists could never have as much impact as Carhart's testimony.

This is why it is so important to document abortionists' public statements. Thanks to the Internet, we can not only find past comments, but we can also be among the first to know when abortionists speak.

One way to keep up on the latest interviews and developments is to sign up for Google News Alerts. This free service is so valuable that we don't know how we ever got along without it. We first learned of the death of Tonya Reaves at a Chicago Planned Parenthood through a Google Alert, and that enabled us to be the first pro-life group to respond. Because of that, we framed the story and pushed it to the national level, forced Planned Parenthood into a defense position, and helped activate other pro-life organizations to join in the call for justice.

Go to www.google.com/newsalerts and input keywords such as abortionist's name, the name of an abortion clinic, or even more general words, such as "abortion" or "RU486" or "Planned Parenthood." The alerts are sent directly to your e-mail in-box. We have dozens of abortion-related topics on Google Alerts that we have set to receive as they appear. It is a great way to stay on top of what is going on by simply checking your e-mail, and it gives you an advantage of being able to respond quickly to breaking abortion-related news.

Learning about a breaking news story or blog entry as it happens can put you into a position to publish your reactions immediately. Often, reporters are looking for reactions or comments on breaking news. If your statement is already out, there is more likelihood that the pro-life perspective will be included in subsequent articles on the topic. Being on top of the news will also help you and your group respond in other ways.

While I was living in San Diego during the Clinton administration, the California Life Coalition monitored any news of the Clintons' next visit to their favorite vacation destination. Because this pro-life group stayed informed, they were able to launch abortion protests at each and every appearance of Bill, Hillary, and Vice President Al Gore in the San Diego area over the entire eight years of Clinton's presidency, often using the opportunity to do media interviews that helped keep the matter of abortion in the public eye.

HOW TO SET UP A GOOGLE NEWS ALERT:

1. Go to Google.com.
2. In the upper right corner of the main search page, click the grid and select the "News" icon.
3. In the search field, type in the key word or phrase you want to track in the news, such as "abortion" or "Florida abortion"; then hit enter or click the magnifying glass at the end of the field.
4. Scroll to the bottom of the search results and click the "Create an email alert for" link.
5. Select the options that best suit your needs and enter your e-mail address.
6. After that, click the red "Create Alert" button and you are done! Links to news articles will begin to arrive in your in-box soon.

27

AT THE ABORTION CLINIC

I prayed for twenty years but received no answer until I prayed with my legs.

—**FREDERICK DOUGLASS**

Another critical means of gathering information is by putting "eyes" on the abortion clinics. The people who spend time outside their local abortion clinics usually know the most about what is going on inside because they see what others don't, and they talk to nearly everyone who is coming and going.

If you are not currently sidewalk counseling, you may want to consider giving it a try. There is nothing quite like the blessing of seeing a woman choose life for her baby and walk away from an abortion appointment because of your encouragement and prayers.

While you are saving lives and helping women, you can become familiar with how the clinic operates. Take the opportunity to talk with vendors who service the abortion clinic. From taxi drivers to trash collectors, these people know things about the clinic that you do not. Ask questions and try to befriend these people to the extent that you are able. You never know when one will drop a critical piece of information that could aid you in bringing abortion to an end in your area.

Make a record of all the vendors you can, and photograph their vehicles, especially if they bear the company logos. This will serve as documentation should you decide to launch a collaborators campaign, which we will discuss later.

Prayer vigils are great opportunities. If you really want to see what is going on at your local clinic, hold a seventy-two-hour round-the-clock prayer vigil, and train everyone to report to you any activity they witness. By doing this, we have documented incidents of illegal activity and medical emergencies that would have gone unnoticed otherwise.

We have discovered that abortion clinics are trending toward evening or late-night abortions or wait until then before they call ambulances for patients who have suffered botched abortions. When there are pro-life eyes on the abortion clinic, it becomes harder for the clinic to hide abortion injuries and deaths.

In fact, the only reason we know about the deaths of women like Christin Gilbert and Jennifer Morbelli, who both died from complications of late-term abortions done by LeRoy Carhart, is because prolifers witnessed incidents and alerted Operation Rescue. Abortionists simply don't self-report abortion-related deaths or injuries! Often they go to great lengths to cover them up. Exposing them can educate the public about abortion dangers, hurt the abortionist's business, and even lead to his or her license revocation.

In Philadelphia, pro-life activists for years generally ignored a seedy west-side abortion clinic known as the Women's Medical Society. They knew a few abortions took place there but thought the numbers were very small compared to other clinics, so they did not maintain a presence there.

The world was shocked to learn in February 2011 that abortionist Kermit Gosnell was operating a busy late-term abortion clinic under the most horrific conditions ever seen.

The police raided Gosnell's clinic under the belief that he was operating a pill mill supplying OxyContin scrips that were sold illicitly on the streets of Philadelphia. What they discovered instead was a "house of horrors," where unlicensed workers drugged pregnant women into stupors and aborted their babies late at night. Most were born alive, only to be killed by Gosnell and his associates, who would stab the newborn infant in the neck with a pair of scissors and clip the struggling baby's spinal cord. Gosnell himself never arrived at the clinic to do these abortions until after eight o'clock in the evening and routinely released the aborted women through the early morning hours with full confidence that pro-life activists were sleeping comfortably in their beds.

Gosnell was later convicted of murdering three newborn babies, although the district attorney indicated in a lengthy grand jury report that literally hundreds of babies were dispatched in this way. Several of Gosnell's employees admitted to snipping newborns' necks as well. We can only wonder how many babies could have been spared if pro-lifers had been aware of his midnight abortion/baby murder operation.

Be observant. Always keep a camera and a notepad with you when you are at the clinic. Take notes and photograph suspicious activity. Even a cell phone camera is good in a pinch. Take pictures to document the arrival of ambulances, building disrepair, overflowing trash, illegal parking, or anything that might potentially be of use. With the advent of digital cameras, there are now no worries about expensive film processing fees, so try to snap more photos than you think you will need.

As previously mentioned, in June 2004, several of our staff and I were praying and sidewalk counseling at George Tiller's late-term abortion clinic in Wichita, Kansas, when an ambulance pulled into the driveway. Cameras in hand, I dashed around to the back of the building to snap photos while Cheryl ran up onto the porch of the pregnancy help center next door to the abortion clinic and began videotaping the ambulance. A gurney was taken inside, then emerged again bearing a woman injured during an abortion. We jumped in our cars and rushed to Wesley Hospital, where Tiller took all his abortion-complication patients. I began snapping the shutter on my digital camera as quickly as it would allow as the gurney was offloaded from the ambulance and pushed through the emergency room doors.

We had just filmed a life-threatening medical emergency from the door of the abortion clinic all the way to the door of the emergency room. It was the best documentation of an abortion emergency that we had ever seen. To top it off, we had captured George Tiller in the act of transporting an injured patient to the emergency room. Because of the photos and video, there was no doubt whatsoever that Tiller and his abortion clinic staff were responsible for sending that poor woman to the hospital.

We enlarged the pictures of Tiller wheeling the injured woman into the emergency room, plastered them on the sides of our Truth Truck, and parked it out in front of his clinic driveway gate, where it aided in turning many women away from having abortions out of concern that they might be next. We put the photos on postcards and sent them to every state legislator, asking for laws to protect women, which helped push forward pro-life legislation. We sent the images to the neighbors of abortion clinic workers, asking them to pray for their neighbor to leave the abortion industry, which prompted several workers to quit their jobs at Tiller's clinic.

Those images helped transform the community sentiment from one that tolerated Tiller's heinous late-term abortion practice to one that actively demanded Tiller be brought to justice. They also informed the legislature of the urgent need for clinic safety standards and accountability.

As noted earlier, we later learned that Tiller had announced his retirement just two weeks before his death. We suspect that he was tossing in the towel so he would not have to face discipline from the Board of Healing Arts. It was that board petition that made Tiller realize that legal actions against him prompted by pro-life supporters were never going to end, and it all started with a few pictures taken by alert pro-lifer activists.

Certainly the success of exposing abortion injuries is not unique to our Wichita project. In Birmingham, savvy pro-lifers photographed emergency workers lifting women out of a run-down abortion mill to gurneys waiting in a trash-strewn ally. The photos, along with the 911 recordings, were widely published by Operation Rescue. We worked with local activists who filed complaints against the New Woman All Women abortion clinic. We had given the Alabama Department of Public Health enough evidence to prompt them to conduct an inspection, which led to the discoveries of deficiencies that filled seventy-six pages. Within four months, the abortion clinic that had operated for over three decades was closed.

Video cameras are important to have on hand as well, especially in the event of an emergency, such as an attack upon you or a fellow pro-lifer, a medical emergency at the clinic, or domestic abuse of a pregnant woman who might not want to go through with an abortion.

While taking a shift outside a Planned Parenthood office in Wilmington, Delaware, in March 2013, Rae Stabosz pulled out her cell phone and began using the video setting, as she had done twice before in the previous weeks, to document a woman being rushed out of the abortion clinic to a waiting ambulance. This time Rae was attacked by a woman and knocked to the ground. Her attacker grabbed Rae's phone and ran into Planned Parenthood. Without a moment's hesitation, Rae, a grandmother of twelve, jumped up and dashed into Planned Parenthood to retrieve her phone, then breathlessly resumed taking the best close-up footage we had ever seen of a woman being loaded into an ambulance, all the while narrating the entire incident.

As she had done before, Rae sent the video to Operation Rescue for publication. The video went viral. News stations, including Fox News' prime-time *Sean Hannity Show*, began to cover the attack and show the video, referring also to the two previous medical emergencies we had published and questioning safety at the abortion clinic. This began to focus attention on Planned Parenthood's shoddy practices, which led to the revelation that there had actually been five botched abortions at that clinic in a three-month time span.

This exposure led two former Planned Parenthood nurses to come forward and publicly describe a "meat market" abortion operation that was so dangerous for women that the nurses had quit in order to preserve their own licenses. This prompted a massive investigation. Abortionist Timothy Liveright and two other workers were fired. The Wilmington Planned Parenthood shut down, along with the Dover location for "cleaning and re-staffing." Delaware would eventually suspend Liveright's medical license because of the danger he posed to the public. Because Planned Parenthood was involved, the story became a national scandal. It was weeks before the clinics could reopen.

The nurses gave powerful testimony during a legislative hearing considering new regulations and oversight for abortion clinics. Serious changes were made in Delaware that we believe will reduce abortions and save lives—all because one grandma had the foresight to pull out her cell phone and hit the button on the video camera.

This is a point we cannot emphasize enough. *Always have a camera on hand!* You never know what is going to happen. You have to be prepared. One of our greatest frustrations is getting calls from activists who report that women were taken away by ambulance, or some other important occurrence, but no one bothered to take a picture to document the incident. At that point, all we have is a story that the abortion clinic can easily deny. Far too many opportunities to report abortion clinics have been lost for this reason.

We must document everything in order to pursue legal action that could close the abortion clinic. *Your camera is your best friend.* DON'T LEAVE HOME WITHOUT IT!

Another important piece of equipment to have on the street is a cell phone. Not only do most cell phones these days have cameras that can take stills or short video clips, but they also provide a critical communications link for you. You can quickly call the police in the event of an emergency, or the media in the event of newsworthy developments. Appointments for abortion-bound women can be arranged on the spot with pro-life centers without having to leave the clinic. In this day and age of free cell phone offers and cheap mobile plans, everyone ministering on the street at abortion clinics should carry a cell phone.

Research and documentation is an ongoing task. Once you have done your homework, gathered background information, and documented wrongdoing, it's time to move on to the next phase in the process of closing an abortion clinic.

HOW TO DOCUMENT A MEDICAL EMERGENCY:

- Make sure you always have a camera that is charged and rapidly accessible.
- Video footage is best, but even cell phone snapshots will work in a pinch.
- Begin to record or snap photos immediately at the onset of an emergency.
- Get as close as you can to the incident, but always remember to stay on public property.
- Make a note of the date and time of the incident, either on a notepad in your pocket or verbally on the video recording.
- Try to take photos that show the context of the incident by trying to get the clinic sign or some other easily identifiable landmark in the photo with the ambulance or emergency responders.
- Photos that show the victim on a gurney being taken from the abortion clinic are useful and dramatic.

- Don't be worried about compromising a patient's privacy when taking photos, because faces can be blurred using editing software before they are published.
- Submit a FOIA request for the 911 audio file and CAD transcript of the call as soon as possible. (See chapter 28.)
- If you do not want to publish the photos and incident report on your own, or even if you do, please send all photos along with your eyewitness account of what happened to Operation Rescue at info.operationrescue@gmail.com with your permission to use your pictures.

28

OPEN RECORDS

Government ought to be all outside and no inside. . . . Everybody knows that corruption thrives in secret places, and avoids public places, and we believe it a fair presumption that secrecy means impropriety.

—**WOODROW WILSON**

Once you have done some background research and become familiarized with the laws, there will probably be additional information you want to get from public agencies. Public records can be obtained through Federal and State Freedom of Information Act (FOIA) requests.

Our good friend Tara Shaver of Project Defending Life in Albuquerque, New Mexico, has uncovered some amazing information using open records requests. She and her husband, Bud, worked for a year as interns for Operation Rescue before moving to Albuquerque with the goal of stopping horrific, late-term abortions there. Once on the ground in Albuquerque, Tara made a broad request for 911 records placed from the city's three abortion clinics: Southwestern Women's Options, Planned Parenthood, and University of New Mexico Reproductive Health Center.

To her surprise, she received more than a dozen 911 recordings and computer-aided dispatch transcripts of abortion-related emergencies that had occurred over the course of the previous twelve months. The content was horrific.

On one emergency call, we could hear a woman moaning and struggling for life. Another indicated that a woman with a previous history of Cesarean-section delivery, who was shockingly thirty-five weeks pregnant, suffered a uterine rupture during her late-term abortion at Southwestern Women's Options. This kind of rupture is life threatening and could kill a woman within minutes.

Tara and Cheryl filed complaints with the New Mexico Medical Board, which is run by a liberal woman named Lynn Hart, who fought to block investigations into the spate of medical emergencies. After applying public pressure Ms. Hart relented and allowed the incidents to be investigated under the caveat that the board—not Tara or Cheryl—would be the official complainant.

The board eventually charged Shelley Sella, the California abortionist and former associate of George Tiller, who flies into Albuquerque to conduct the latest of abortions. She was accused of gross negligence for ignoring the patient's medical history of a previous C-section, which made the client a high risk for complications if labor was induced. Sella used Cytotec, an ulcer drug that causes very strong and unpredictable contractions, in an outpatient setting to induce labor. Those contractions were so strong that they broke open the woman's uterus and thrust part of her baby into her abdominal cavity.

After a three-day disciplinary trial, the board inexcusably cleared Sella of wrongdoing, but not before the case became front-page news. The coverage fostered new public discussion and awareness of the horrific nature and questionable morality of late-term abortions. No one could have bought that kind of publicity! Even though the outcome was not what we hoped, there were major benefits from the case all the same. It was a huge step in the right direction, all because of information discovered through an open records request.

In Kansas, another open records request made by our office helped shine the light on political corruption and cowardice.

After years of investigation, while serving terms as Kansas attorney general and Johnson County district attorney, pro-life prosecutor Phill Kline filed a massive 107-count criminal case against Planned Parenthood, alleging they had performed illegal abortions and manufactured evidence to cover their crimes. Kline was replaced in the DA's office by a supposedly pro-life Republican, Steve Howe, who inherited the case from Kline.

However, Howe was a political enemy of Kline's who lacked the will to prosecute. The case had gone up on an appeal to the Kansas Supreme Court, which was dominated by appointees of radical former governor Kathleen Sebelius, who would later serve as US Health and Human Services secretary in the Obama administration. Howe was content to let the case atrophy until the court could rule. After several months, the court finally remanded the case back to Howe for prosecution.

Kline's investigation had originated during his term as attorney general, when he opened an inquisition related to abortion clinics under the supervision of Shawnee District court judge Richard Anderson, who maintained the inquisition files.

Howe began dismissing the case against Planned Parenthood one group of charges at a time. He claimed his decisions to dismiss the charges were made in conjunction with fellow Republican Derek Schmidt, who also ran for office as a pro-life supporter. They determined that the documents that were the basis for Kline's charges had all been destroyed, and so the prosecution could not go forward.

We were disturbed by this because it seemed obvious that Judge Anderson would have a pristine copy of the evidence in his possession. In fact, Sebelius-appointed attorney general Steve Six had even at one time procured a gag order against Anderson that blocked him from releasing the very files in question. There had been heavy media coverage of that, of which Howe and Schmidt were well aware.

We decided to use an open records request to find the answer. We asked Judge Anderson, not for the files themselves, but for any documentation of the files' location. In his denial of the documents, Anderson revealed two very important points.

First, he indicated that the files, which had been in his custody for years, had been transferred to the custody of the Shawnee County clerk of the court. This was evidence that the records were not destroyed, as Howe and Schmidt had led everyone to believe, but were safely in the court's custody.

Second, Anderson said that there was no record that anyone had ever made formal inquiry about the records, and no record to show that anyone had ever requested to inspect them!

These were bombshell revelations! Had the Planned Parenthood case been dismissed based on a falsehood? We thought so and filed ethics complaints against District Attorney Howe and Attorney General Schmidt, which, as of this writing, are still open cases. We still maintain that the Planned Parenthood case was prosecutable and that the open records request had uncovered political corruption inside the Republican Party, which was more interested in discrediting its political rival, Phill Kline, than enforcing the law.

Capable of uncovering everything from abortion abuses to pro-abortion political obstructionism, the open record request is a valuable tool that every pro-life activist should know how to use.

Open records laws vary from state to state, so be sure you are familiar with those in your state before trying to file a request. Remember, open records requests apply only to government agencies and not to private businesses.

Following are some of the kinds of things you can obtain from open records requests:

- Medical license applications and disciplinary documents
- Business license information
- 990 federal tax forms for nonprofit businesses (for-profit businesses are exempt)
- Court records and documents (criminal and civil)
- Health and safety inspection reports
- 911 recordings and computer-aided dispatch transcripts
- Autopsy reports
- Statistical data related to abortion, maintained by most state health departments
- Communications between government workers/office holders, including e-mails, receipts, meeting logs, etc.
- Military history

Many open records are very easy to get. Some are kept online, so there is no need to ask for them.

Be sure to check the website of the agency from which you are seeking open records, and see if it has a procedure for obtaining open records. Sometimes there is an e-mail address that will accept requests and return the documents to you in electronic form. Whatever the case, follow the directions given to maximize your chances of getting what you want with minimum hassle.

Some requests for records will need to be made in writing. In that case, letters should be sent certified with delivery confirmation. You will then have proof of the date the letter was sent, and you will receive a card in the mail confirming that the letter was received and who signed for it. All this is important information in the event the agency is nonresponsive or resists giving you records to which you know you are legally entitled.

If an agency fails to answer within the time allowed by statute, make sure you follow up with a second request. In the event the agency is still nonresponsive, you may be eligible to sue them for the records. Most states provide for attorney fees to be awarded in the event that a requesting party prevails in court, which makes it a bit easier to find an attorney to help.

We have worked with three pro-life attorney groups, the Thomas More Society in Chicago, Alliance Defending Freedom, and Life Legal Defense Foundation, when we have needed extra help with open records requests. They have both been very helpful and have offered their services at no charge to us.

In making open records requests, we have found that we get better results if we make the requests as individuals and not as representatives of any group. When some records custodians realize you are asking for information related to abortion, they become suspicious and unhelpful.

Probably one of the most common and important reasons for making an open records request will be in the event of a medical emergency at an abortion clinic. You will want to make a request for the 911 records as soon as possible.

The release of such records can actually lead to the closure of an abortion clinic, as it did in Birmingham, Alabama, in 2012. Pro-life activists photographed two ambulances at the New Woman All Women abortion clinic on January 21, 2012, picking up two abortion patients who were then transported to a local hospital. But they didn't stop there. They sought and obtained the 911 call, which was placed by clinic owner Diane Derzis. She was heard admitting that the patients had been overmedicated by a clinic worker. Complaints were filed and the health department, which documented the fact that the clinic was a repeat offender, ordered the clinic to close. The 911 recording was a critical piece of evidence in that case.

First, determine who maintains the emergency communications in your area. Good places to start looking are the local police department, sheriff's office, fire department, or county office of emergency communications. It varies from one jurisdiction to another. It is important to make your request to the proper agency.

There are some very definite dos and don'ts for making a request for emergency communications.

DO make your request as soon as possible after the incident. Some counties delete the 911 recordings after a year, some in less time than that.

DO specify the address where the call originated and approximate date and time of the incident.

DO be prepared to pay a modest fee for the records, although often the records can be obtained free of charge, especially if they can be sent via e-mail.

DON'T elaborate on the nature of the incident. Just ask for records pertaining to all calls placed from a specific address on a certain date or date range.

DON'T be so specific that you do not get what you want. For example, if you ask for a call placed at 10:00 a.m., and the call was actually placed at 9:45 a.m., you might not receive the records at all.

DON'T mention the word *abortion* or the clinic's name. This raises red flags and gives staff an excuse to deny your request.

DON'T mention that you are a pro-life supporter or that you represent any group. It is best to make the request as an individual citizen.

Public records are just that—public. However, it is legal for some information to be redacted (deleted), especially if it is personal in nature, such as social security numbers or home addresses. Over-redaction can sometimes be a problem, but any record is better than no record. There are remedies if a record is redacted to the point that it is concealing information to which you are legally entitled, but you may need to contact an attorney.

Here is a sample request for 911 records using fictitious information. Please use whatever information is applicable to your situation.

January 1, 2012

Office of Emergency Communications
124 E. Main Street
Anytown, California 92071

Dear Records Custodian:

This is a request for public records under the FOIA and the state's open records law.

Please send me copies of all recordings of 911 emergency communications placed from 345 N. First Ave., Anytown, California, 92072, for December 20–25, 2011. I am also asking for all Computer-Aided Dispatch Transcripts related to the call or calls.

I would appreciate it if the records could be sent in digital format to me at the following e-mail address:

janedoe@abc.com

If that is not possible, please mail the records to:

Jane Doe
P.O. Box 1234
Anytown, California 92017
(619) 555-1234

Thank you very much for your time and attention to this request.

Sincerely,

Jane Doe

Notice that there is nothing in the request that would raise any concerns or relate the request to abortion in any way. Sometimes, however, records custodians will call and ask why you want the records. In reality, it is none of their business, but in practicality, you need to have a generic answer ready that will appease them.

Among our favorites is to inform the custodian that we need the records for research. Whatever you decide to tell them, it is best to omit any reference to abortion or your pro-life work. Abortion is a politically charged subject that evokes strong emotions. These records are so important that we simply cannot risk a pro-abortion clerk denying our requests based on our pro-life beliefs. That has been known to happen. It's best to simply leave the "A" word out of your open records requests.

29

THE CONFIDENTIAL INFORMANT

When law enforcement and whistleblowers threaten their corrupt allies, they change the rules of the game.

—**HOWARD DEAN**

It is not uncommon for those inside the abortion industry to contact pro-life groups with information. They do it for a variety of reasons. Some are guilt-ridden about their work and want to unburden themselves. Some do it to right a wrong. Whatever their motivation, these informants can be a valuable source of information.

If people know you seek information, they will seek you out.

Such was the case in 2012 when a woman named Deborah Edge contacted us with information about a late-term abortionist in Houston, Texas. She had worked for Douglas Karpen for almost fifteen years. She received one of our flyers explaining our Abortion Whistleblowers Program, which had been sent to every abortion clinic in the United States. She smuggled the flyer out of the clinic and made the call.

What we learned from her was stunning. Over the course of several months, more and more details of a horrific, late-term abortion practice emerged. Women were slapped for slow compliance, heavy women were called names and treated rudely, and babies were routinely born alive, only to have their heads twisted or crushed as they struggled for life.

Deborah persuaded three other Karpen employees to come forward. In December 2012, Gigi Aguilar e-mailed Cheryl photos of a late-term baby that had been aborted. Those pictures changed everything.

The baby was huge, with pink skin, brown hair, and open hazel eyes. He was so big that it struck the ladies working at the clinic, and Gigi took photos with her cell phone. The little boy's neck bore a large, ragged gash, consistent with tearing that might occur if his head had been forcefully twisted. Gigi indicated that she believed the baby was twenty-six weeks, but he could have been older.

The legal limit for abortions in Texas is twenty-four weeks. We knew we had just been given evidence of a crime, perhaps even murder, but we were still unclear if the baby in the photo had been born alive, so we passed them on to attorneys with the Alliance Defending Freedom, a pro-life legal organization that was helping to represent the women who had come forward.

Then we received a second set of photos. This baby was also huge and had the same ragged gash at the neck. Working with pro-life physicians and using a photo of a baby's foot in an adult hand, we roughly estimated that the second baby may have been between twenty-six and thirty weeks gestation—clearly beyond the legal limit in Texas.

The case was disturbingly similar to the criminal case against Kermit Gosnell, the West Philadelphia abortionist who was about to go on trial for murdering babies born alive at his squalid late-term abortion mill. There were almost identical allegations, including untrained workers providing services for which they were not qualified, reused disposable surgical equipment, falsification of ultrasound results in order to manipulate fetal ages, and illegal late-term abortions. The photos added the possibility that Karpen, like Gosnell, was committing murder on newborn babies.

An Alliance Defending Freedom (ADF) attorney forwarded the photos to the investigator at the Texas Medical Board. We understood that if there had been criminal conduct, it would be the board's duty to report it to the appropriate authorities.

Instead, we were shocked to receive a letter from the TMB in February 2013, closing the complaint against Karpen. The letter read in part:

> The investigation referenced above has been dismissed because the Board determined there was insufficient evidence to prove that a violation of the Medical Practices Act occurred. Specifically, this investigation determined that Dr. Karpen did not violate the laws connected with the practice of medicine and there is no evidence of inappropriate behavior, therefore no further action will be taken.

How in the world could anyone look at the photos of those poor babies and say there was "no evidence of inappropriate behavior"? We were stunned! Had someone gotten to the board? Had there been some political interference that led to this inexplicable result?

We simply couldn't let this be the last word.

We had wanted to interview our Karpen informants on video, to have a record of their stories, but we were shorthanded and swamped at the office and unable to finalize arrangements. After we received the TMB dismissal letter, getting the interviews seemed even more important. By now, Cheryl was about to fly off to Philadelphia to attend and report on the Kermit Gosnell murder trial. I called Mark Crutcher, who lives in Texas, to see if he could help.

While Cheryl was in Philadelphia, arrangements were made for Mark to travel to Houston to interview three of the former Karpen employees, Deborah Edge, Gigi Aguilar, and Krystal Rodriguez. By the time he actually conducted the interviews on May 3, the Gosnell case was on jury watch.

Ten days later, Gosnell was convicted on three counts of first-degree murder for snipping the necks of newborn babies, one count of involuntary manslaughter related to the overdose death of patient Karnamaya Mongar, and more than two hundred other abortion and corruption-related crimes.

Then late the following day, Life Dynamics Inc. released the first fourteen-minute interview with the three whistle-blowers. Operation Rescue followed up the next morning with a complete exposé that included the full-color photos of the two babies and called for a criminal prosecution.

Texas Lt. Governor David Dewhurst issued a statement the following afternoon demanding a full-scale investigation into the practices of Houston abortionist Douglas Karpen. The news broke nationwide and was featured for two days on the Drudge Report. Our phones rang off the hook.

In Washington, DC, Rep. Trent Franks (R-AZ) announced that he would amend his bill, the District of Columbia Pain Capable Unborn Child Protection Act (H.R. 1797), to apply nationwide. He led a hearing on the legislation in the US House Committee of the Judiciary Subcommittee on the Constitution and Civil Justice, where he showed the photos of the Karpen babies taken directly from our website. The hearing was streamed live on the Internet.

While as of this writing it is unclear whether Douglas Karpen will ever be brought to justice, the information given to us by our four informants has already had a huge impact on the abortion debate in America. Their courage in coming forward caused influencers such as news reporters, bloggers, and legislators to refocus on the rampant abuses that take place daily at our nation's abortion clinics and on the question of whether this is really how we want to treat each other as human beings.

We are grateful for the day when Deborah Edge rang our phone, and we are always expectant of the next informant to bring forth information damaging to the abortion cartel that will rock the nation.

Operation Rescue makes it very clear that we are constantly seeking information about abortion abuses. We widely advertise that we offer a twenty-five-thousand-dollar reward through our Abortion Whistle-blowers Program for information leading to the arrest and conviction of abortionists who are breaking the law. We regularly send flyers with details of our program to every abortion clinic in the country. Because of that, we work with many confidential informants, some who are still working at clinics or who have access to current inside information.

Most informants do not want anyone to know they are talking to us. We take the confidentiality of informants seriously and do everything we can to protect their identities. That helps them trust us and it keeps the information flowing.

I have a saying about such informants: "Trust, but verify." Sometimes people who want to give you information simply cannot be trusted. When an informant first contacts us, we take the time to check the person's background to make sure she (or he) is who she represents herself to be. A Google search is wise, but if there is a need for additional caution, background-checking services such as BeenVerified can also be useful.

We carefully interview our informants, usually multiple times, and attempt to build relationships with them. We independently verify as many facts as we can. For example, suppose the informant indicates that a certain abortionist has been involved in a malpractice suit. That information can be easily confirmed through a search of court records on the Internet. Independent verification can help you determine how much trust to place in the information the informant is providing.

These conversations are almost always recorded. In some cases, the informant may feel that he or she has sufficiently unburdened after the first interview, and cuts off all communication. In that case, you will be very glad to have a recording of that conversation, especially if it contains information about specific abortion abuses or criminal activity that can be verified by authorities.

It is critical that informants are encouraged to provide as much documentation as they can. The following story proves it.

In Kansas, during the radically pro-abortion Sebelius administration, an intense effort to investigate abortion clinics was under way. Pro-life attorney general Phill Kline routinely made headlines in his effort to bring abortionists such as George Tiller and Planned Parenthood to justice. This abortion battle played out through wildly contentious political campaigns. As mentioned in chapter 11, in 2006, Tiller and his political action committee dumped an estimated $1 million under the table into defeating Kline. Sebelius herself hand-picked Paul Morrison, who promised to stop the investigations, to oppose Kline. Kline was mercilessly vilified in mailings and television ads in an attempt to scare voters away from him. The scare tactic worked. Kline was defeated as attorney general, but was immediately appointed to the office of Johnson County district attorney, where he then pursued a case against Planned Parenthood for committing illegal abortions and manufacturing evidence to cover it up. The Sebelius administration continued to aggressively block Kline's investigations and vilify him in the media.

During this tumultuous time, I received an unexpected phone call from a woman named Tina David who had recently left employment with Tiller. We knew she was the real deal because we had frequently seen her at the clinic. Tina wanted to talk. I invited her to our office, where we interviewed her and taped the conversation.

Tina told us all about her work at Tiller's late-term abortion clinic and about the stress it put her under. She literally couldn't sleep at night after what she experienced there.

At one point, Tina began talking about a big party she had attended at the governor's mansion while Tiller was still under active criminal investigation. That piqued our attention. She told us that Governor Sebelius had invited Tiller and his entire abortion clinic staff to a special dinner at Cedar Crest, the governor's official residence, for a lavish party to honor Tiller. Tina described how they were treated to steak and lobster, and got a chance to hobnob with the governor.

"I'd give my eyeteeth for a picture of that," said Cheryl, knowing the information was useless without documentation of some kind.

"Oh, I have pictures! You can have them," Tina responded.

After the interview, Cheryl took the former abortion worker home, where Tina gave her a Walmart CD containing twenty-seven photos taken during that party at Cedar Crest, including photographs of Sebelius holding up a campaign T-shirt bearing her name and Paul Morrison's, while pointing to Tiller in acknowledgment. We immediately made an open records request to the governor's office for documents related to the soiree, being careful not to let them know exactly who we were, what we were after, or why.

In response to that request, we received receipts and evidence that Sebelius's party for Tiller's staff was paid for with state tax dollars. Sebelius tried to deny it and contrived several different excuses to explain the event, but the photos and other documents were irrefutable.

We broke the story. Those photos revealed Sebelius's deep connections and friendship with Tiller and her willingness to shield him from criminal prosecution at a time when he was an active suspect in an illegal late-term abortion case. It was a scandal that ultimately delayed Sebelius's confirmation as secretary of health and human services for weeks, and very nearly tanked her nomination altogether.

Elsewhere, in Iowa, California, and Texas, former Planned Parenthood administrators and officers have come forward with information about illegal billing practices. In all three states, suits have been filed by ADF under federal whistle-blower laws that are exposing massive fraud perpetrated on taxpayers and patients.

These whistle-blowers are valuable assets that can bring down abortion businesses and even land abortionists in jail.

In 2007, Massachusetts abortionist Rapin Osathanondh killed Laura Hope Smith during an abortion. An untrained receptionist was the only other worker present in the office at the time of Laura's abortion. Operation Rescue was contacted by Laura's mother, Eileen. We worked to file complaints with the medical board and pressure the state attorney for a criminal prosecution.

During this time, Kim, the employee who had witnessed Laura's death, came forward and became friendly with Eileen. She eventually cooperated with the medical board's investigation, telling them that Osathanondh had no working emergency equipment, which would have been necessary to save Laura's life. According to Kim's sworn testimony, after Laura died, Osathanondh purchased the emergency equipment and backdated the records to make it appear that it was on hand before Laura's fatal appointment.

Because of Kim's brave testimony, Osathanondh was forced to surrender his medical license, close his two abortion offices, and formally promise to never again seek licensure in any state. Kim's testimony was also the basis for manslaughter charges against Osathanondh, who eventually pled guilty and was sentenced to six months in jail. Kim was the recipient of Operation Rescue's first twenty-five-thousand-dollar reward under the Abortion Whistleblower's Program.

Many times informants are taking great risks to blow the whistle on the abortion cartel, and they need to be treated with respect and friendship. When dealing with these people, it is important to have a support structure in place for them. Have legal assistance at the ready, as well as resources that can provide financial aid and employment placement assistance, if necessary. It is also important to provide spiritual support for them as well, especially if they are in the process of transitioning out of the abortion industry.

If all this seems overwhelming, Operation Rescue is willing to work with pro-life activists and groups to assist in managing informants and to ensure that the information supplied by them gets into the right hands.

TIPS FOR DEALING WITH A CONFIDENTIAL INFORMANT:

- Try to build a relationship of trust.
- Handle the person with love and compassion. He or she deserves to be treated with respect.
- If possible, record your initial conversation in case the informant never contacts you again.
- Attempt to independently verify the information you receive, to corroborate its veracity.
- Get as much documentation as you can from the informant, including photos that support his or her claims.
- If the informant requires that his or her identity remain confidential, diligently honor that request.
- If legal issues arise, consult a pro-life attorney.
- If your informant supplies you with evidence of criminal conduct, report it to the police.
- Advise the informant of Operation Rescue's Abortion Whistleblowers Program, which offers a reward for information leading to the arrest and conviction of abortionists who are breaking the law.
- Never give an informant money up front, because that could damage the person's credibility if his or her testimony is ever required. If the informant is in dire need, offer referrals to other groups or agencies who can help in that way.

30

THE STING

Opportunities multiply as they are seized. —**SUN TZU**

It's not very difficult to get abortion clinic staff to admit wrongdoing. The trick is to get them to make the incriminating admissions on tape. That brings us to the topic of what we call the "abortion sting." This tactic has been made popular in recent years with YouTube and some national press.

However, Operation Rescue has been conducting similar stings for years. Using this tactic, we have caught abortion clinic workers admitting that they are willing to conceal child rape, unlicensed workers illegally practicing medicine, and even evidence of an elaborate, bi-state late-term-abortion scheme.

We recently conducted a six-month sting operation on infamous late-term abortionist James Scott Pendergraft IV, using the undercover call that we discussed earlier. Pendergraft is a particularly troubled Florida abortionist who runs a chain of five abortion clinics in the

Orlando area. His medical license has been suspended four times, and he was recently ordered to pay a whopping $37 million to a former abortion patient ten years after a failed abortion left her baby seriously injured and handicapped.

Pendergraft launched LateTermAbortion.net, a clandestine late-term abortion scheme that he operated in "the Washington D.C., Northern Virginia and Maryland area." Pendergraft offers to provide fetal injections to women in the latest stages of pregnancy that will kill the baby. The woman then has the option of delivering her dead baby at Pendergraft's secret abortion clinic, or returning to her home state for the delivery at a hospital of her choice.

"Once the fetal heart beat has stopped, the process of removing the fetus from the mother's womb is no longer defined as an abortion," states Pendergraft on his website's "Frequently Asked Questions" page. He offers this as a way to force hospitals and physicians that otherwise may balk at abortion to finish the abortion process since the woman now faces a serious life-threatening condition.

Pro-life supporters were appalled at Pendergraft's brazen willingness to endanger the lives and health of women in order to make a political point, but so much secrecy surrounded his operation that no one knew where his clinic was or who he was working with, even months after Pendergraft launched his predatory website.

We decided the sting was the best way to discover Pendergraft's illegal operation and expose him and his accomplice. I called Pendergraft, posing as the husband of a woman who wanted a late-term abortion after her own physician refused to do it. I was apparently quite convincing, since Pendergraft seemed unguarded and was incredibly open and talkative. In all, we recorded over three hours of conversations with Pendergraft, during which he described the abortion process, detailed the payment procedure (cash is wired to his Florida bank account), and documented his promises to fly from Florida to

Maryland to meet prospective customers on less than a day's notice to escort them to the abortion clinic, where they would benefit from his twenty-five years of experience.

We discovered that Pendergraft was working in Maryland (where he holds no active medical license), with abortionist Harold O. Alexander, who runs an abortion clinic in Forestville, Maryland. Alexander was already in hot water with the state medical board, which had charged him with a number of shocking allegations, including "sexual boundary" violations, botched abortions, shoddy or nonexistent record keeping, and the illegal prescribing of large amounts of Viagra and other drugs to himself and non-patients.

We kept the information quiet to avoid tipping off the abortionists while we filed our complaints against Pendergraft and Alexander and waited for the board to do its job. We had hoped that board investigators would catch them in the act of providing dangerous and illegal late-term abortions. Eventually, we made information obtained through this sting public.

Alexander admitted that he was involved in Pendergraft's late-term abortion scheme and was formally charged by the board with destroying related abortion records that were under subpoena. Alexander's medical license was suspended, and we obtained assurances from the Maryland Board of Physicians that Pendergraft's dangerous late-term abortion scheme had been terminated.

Another popular way to conduct a sting is to send a team into the clinic with a hidden video camera. This type of elaborate hoax scenario was made famous by Lila Rose of Live Action, who has surreptitiously videotaped abortion clinic workers and providers saying the darnedest things. This requires a team that is good at role-playing, as well as specialized video cameras that are undetectable during the personal interview. We have used cameras that look like ballpoint pens and small "spy" cameras that can be hidden in a purse. Such equipment is easy to get on the Internet but takes some practice to master.

Holding to the model that "simple is better," we suggest the undercover call as the most efficient way to conduct a sting, especially for those just getting started. There are audio recording devices that allow you to hook up a digital recorder directly to your handset. Perhaps the easiest way, however, is to simply put the phone on speaker and place the recorder near the speaker.

Before you make the call, think about the information you want to know. It may be helpful to make notes or write down questions to ask. If calling to make an abortion appointment, think about the character you will be playing during the call and prepare by determining your character's age, date of birth, date of last menstrual period, a phone number that would be local to the clinic, and circumstances in your character's life that will help you carry off the part, always remembering the adage that "simple is better."

Never let the abortion workers know they've been the subject of a sting until the information has already been made public. This will allow you to continue to mine the unsuspecting clinic workers for information and will prevent them from publicizing their own spin ahead of your story. It's best to keep the abortion clinics on the defense.

There is only one thing better than catching abortion clinic employees making ridiculous statements, and that is catching them making incriminating statements. You never really know what these people will say to you, but they may say it only once, so be sure to record the conversations and archive them for future reference.

When releasing audio recordings that contain no video, such as 911 calls or files from a digital audio recorder, it's a good idea to produce a video using the recording as the soundtrack. Video simply gets more attention in this visual age of ours.

You don't need fancy software or expertise. Such videos are easy to produce on your computer. Windows Movie Maker comes free on Windows computers and is pretty easy to use. Make a folder and save the photos or video clips you might want to use to illustrate your recording, then drag them into the Windows Movie Maker or other video editing program.

Animation features can zoom in or pan across still photos to add visual interest, but try to limit your use of fancy special effects, because they tend to make videos appear homemade instead of professional. We recommend that your videos not be more than four or five minutes, with three minutes being a comfortable length for most viewers. If the audio is even remotely difficult to hear, consider adding subtitles to help make the message easier to understand. Make sure to put your organization's name and website at the end to draw new readers and increase your effectiveness.

If you have a budget for it, you can have your video professionally produced, but be forewarned that it can be pricey. However, it may be worth it depending on what you are trying to accomplish. Just know there are options, and they may not have to cost you a "pretty penny" to be effective.

When you are happy with your production, upload it to YouTube, Vimeo, or other video sharing sites; then post a link wherever you can, including on Facebook, Twitter, and other social networking sites, in addition to your own website and e-mail list. The more people who have the opportunity to view your evidence, the more impact you will have.

For examples of dozens of videos of this nature, please visit Operation Rescue's YouTube channel at http://www.youtube.com/user/cherylsullenger/featured.

TIPS FOR PRODUCING A VIDEO FOR INTERNET-SHARING SITES:

- Set up accounts on as many video-sharing sites as possible. This will increase visibility for your video.
- Before you begin, gather all the video, audio, and photo files you plan to use into one computer folder. This will save you time later in the editing process.
- Whatever materials you use in producing your video, if you do not own them, make sure you have permission to use them.
- Try to make your video as brief as possible. The shorter it is, the greater the likelihood that people will take the time to watch it. (Between one and three minutes is ideal in most cases.)
- Edit out long periods of video or audio where nothing is happening.
- Put your organization's name and website at the end of the video. This can increase your visibility and help news organizations find you if the video is newsworthy.
- After publishing your video, post it to your blog or website and share it on your social networking sites. Issue a press release with a link to it, if appropriate.

31

GETTING THE MESSAGE PAST THE GATEKEEPERS

Truth at last cannot be hidden. —**LEONARDO DA VINCI**

Once you have documented the "dirt" on your local abortion clinic, it is critical that you get this information into the public's hands. This is a crucial aspect of closing abortion clinics, and in this day and age of electronics media and the twenty-four-hour news cycle, getting the word out has never been easier.

However, there are those who resist the pro-life message, especially if it documents abortion abuses. Prosecuting attorneys may not want to prosecute an abortionist because they think it might be damaging to their careers. Boards may not want to discipline abortionists because of a political climate that favors abortion. News organizations hesitate to cover stories of abortion abuses because editorial boards are generally friendly to the pro-abortion position. Some news organizations go so far as to serve as de facto propaganda organs for the abortion cartel. The challenge is to bypass the gatekeepers who cover up for abortion clinics, and get the message out in spite of them.

How you do this really depends on how the information can best be used to accomplish your goals.

On the most basic level, let's suppose you have amassed a stack of malpractice suits, disciplinary action documents, and/or health department deficiency reports that pertain to your local abortion clinic. The people who need that information most are the women who have scheduled appointments there. Brochures detailing the sordid details are effective tools that can help women understand the dangers of abortion and save lives in the short term.

We did just that in San Diego, most notably with an abortionist named Robert Santella. We created brochures detailing his disciplinary history, and sidewalk counselors handed them out to abortion-bound women outside his clinic.

We told them of patient Judy L., whose care for surgical complications was delayed by Santella as he ran personal errands instead of getting to the hospital and treating his patient, and of Cheryl L., who was forced to wait in pain for over twenty-five hours after being admitted to a local hospital before Santella bothered to see or treat her. We described the horrific case of Randa P., whose wanted baby was stillborn because Santella inadequately monitored her pregnancy and failed to recognize symptoms that were obvious warning signs. We warned women that Santella routinely failed to perform adequate testing on women before surgeries and that his record keeping was so poor that it constituted unprofessional conduct.

Many women decided wisely against abortions after being provided with this important information. Our research was saving lives.

The information gathered can have a longer-term effect if it is used to influence public opinion. Reference your documentation when writing letters to editors, legislators, and other decision makers. Proper documentation of abortion abuses has been foundational to passing pro-life laws in many states and in changing public attitudes about abortion.

Because of the pro-abortion bias of the mainstream media, we have been forced to learn how to get our story into the news in spite of media bias, how to strategically plant information with friendly media, and how to sidestep those who cover up for abortionists, all by turning our social networking accounts into pro-life educational outreaches that can reach millions.

A great example of that was in the case of Kermit Gosnell. For the first three weeks of his trial, as some of the most horrific testimony ever given against an abortionist was being heard day after day, only about three local news outlets were covering the story. The case was every bit as salacious, if not more so, as some of the other murder cases that were getting wall-to-wall news coverage.

When Cheryl began attending the trial on the first day of week three, the seats in the courtroom were mostly empty. She was the only one posting stories from the courtroom from a pro-life perspective. Her writing got a lot of attention inside the pro-life movement, but it also raised questions about why the national media was absent.

I spoke with Bryan Kemper of Stand True about the dearth of coverage, and we decided to launch a *tweetfest* using the hashtag "#Gosnell" to demand media coverage. We promoted the tweetup on Facebook and linked back to Cheryl's stories. The hashtag allowed everyone commenting on the Gosnell trial to be able to see everyone else's tweets posted under the same hashtag.

The overwhelming response completely blew us away.

More than ten thousand people signed up on Facebook to participate, but that was just the beginning. "#Gosnell" trended in the number one spot on Twitter for a day and a half. J.D. Mullane, a local columnist at PhillyBurbs.com, secretly snapped a photo of the rows of empty seats in the courtroom, reserved for media that never showed up, then posted it to Twitter, including @OperationRescue in the body of his tweet. That photo became the image that defined the message. Thousands of times the question was asked: "Where is the national media?"

The Monday after the tweetup, Cheryl was in court to see the previously empty courtroom crowded with reporters from every major news organization. The tweetup had literally shamed the national media into covering the trial. Press conferences and prayer vigils outside the court punctuated the effort. By the time closing arguments were given, the courtroom was packed. Later, Fox News aired a one-hour special on the Gosnell trial called "See No Evil," that was so favorable to the pro-life cause that it could have been written by my staff!

The tweetup had successfully bypassed the gatekeepers to reach the grass roots and thereby forced the story into the national media.

DECIPHERING TWITTER SHORTHAND FOR THE BEGINNER

Twitter = name of a popular social networking site.

tweet = a post on Twitter. Posts are limited to 142 characters, including spaces.

= hashtag. A hashtag allows your post to appear in a searchable stream of tweets with the same hashtag. For example, searching #prolife on Twitter will produce a stream of tweets under that hashtag. Some people use hashtags to cleverly convey a point, such as #BestIdeaEver. Words or phrases after a hashtag should contain no spaces or hyphens.

RT = Retweet. When this appears in a tweet, it means that it is a repost that originated with another user.

MT = Modified Tweet. This is a user reposting a slight rewording of someone else's tweet.

DM = Direct Message. This function of Twitter allows you to communicate privately with another user.

@ = at. Putting this symbol before a user's screen name, such as @ OperationRescue, will "tag" that user and allow your tweet to post in his home stream. This is also called a "mention."

Tweetfest (or, tweetup) = refers to an effort to get large numbers of people to tweet under a common hashtag.

trending = a word, phrase, or hashtag that is being heavily used at a given time. Campaigns are often launched to get a particular subject trending, increasing the visibility of that subject on Twitter.

32

EFFECTIVE PRESS RELEASES

Without publicity, no good is permanent; under the auspices of publicity, no evil can continue.

—**JEREMY BENTHAM, 1768**

Whenever abortion is in the news, it is good for the pro-life cause. Our job is to make sure abortion stays in the headlines, and a press release is one very effective way to do it. We have two goals when publishing press releases.

First, we want to encourage pro-life supporters. Anytime there is good news, it should be shared. Even modest successes can be promoted as big steps forward for the cause. We have found that pro-life activists spend a lot of time dwelling on how far we have to go and not enough time celebrating how far we have come. We all need encouragement. We all need to know that somehow, somewhere, activists just like you and me are winning significant battles against the abortion "Goliath." We need to be reminded that we can win. Your successes can serve to encourage and inspire others to press forward. Do everything you can to give them hope that victory is right around the corner, because it is.

Second, we use our press releases to discourage and dishearten the enemy. The pro-abortion side is already a dejected bunch. One needs only to read their blogs and occasional editorials. They know they are losing, and they don't know what to do about it. They are angry, frustrated, and discouraged. There is an emotional and psychological aspect to what we are doing. If those on the other side get so discouraged that they begin to look for another line of work, that is a victory for us. They need to see optimism and energy from us. They need to believe that we are winning and they are losing and that they are just one short step away from utter defeat. Do what you can to take away their hope in the abortion cause with news of your victories.

In 2006 we filed a complaint with the Kansas State Board of Healing Arts against late-term abortionist George Tiller and his associate, Ann Kristin Neuhaus, whom we discussed previously. Because of urgent developments in other projects, that complaint went to the back of our minds. Tiller was criminally charged and went to trial in March 2009. Of course, our press releases flew out the door during that time, but there was no lack of media attention. The street outside the courthouse was lined with satellite trucks from every imaginable news outlet, and each morning there was a line outside the courtroom door of folks hoping to get a seat. But when Tiller was acquitted, I have to admit, it looked a little bleak.

However, just moments after the verdict, the Kansas State Board of Healing Arts released a press statement announcing that it had charged Tiller with eleven counts based on our complaint. We immediately dropped a press release whose headline screamed, "It's Not Over: Tiller Charged With 11 Counts By KSBHA. Tiller could still lose his medical license." We were not defeated! In fact, we were back on the offensive, and we used our press release to make sure everyone knew it.

The fact is that the KSBHA petition against Tiller had been pending for months. Only after his acquittal did the board make it public. Their press release and ours took the wind out of the sails of Tiller's pro-abortion supporters.

A few months later, abortionist Shelley Sella gave an interview to MSNBC where she made the following insightful statement referring to the announcement that the KSBHA was pursuing action against Tiller and its impact on him: "[Tiller] didn't even have time to enjoy the fact that he had finally won. And then, another blow. It was just never going to end."

This was a perfect example of how a press release can discourage those who support abortion and encourage those who support life.

Dropping an effective press release can also result in interviews that can potentially broadcast your message out to millions of people. There are several things you can do to make sure your press releases get in the right hands and are taken seriously.

Whether you are breaking a hot story or commenting on breaking news, the content of your press release should be newsworthy. There's truth to the old news idiom that says that "Dog bites man" isn't newsworthy, but "Man bites dog"—now, that's news. Look for ways to make your release fit into the "Man bites dog" category.

One of our favorite headlines was "La Quinta Sends Tiller Packing." It was a clever play on words. As we mentioned in chapter 7, we were successful at terminating the La Quinta Inn's business arrangement that allowed George Tiller to use the hotel as a functional part of his late-term abortion clinic in Wichita, Kansas. After carefully documenting the relationship, we took it to the La Quinta corporate staff, who put a halt to the arrangement, which posed a danger to the lives and health of women and gave the corporation name a black eye. Our headline made La Quinta the hero and Tiller the villain in one pithy statement.

Tying a local news event to a national news story can give your release extra attention. Here are some examples.

Each January, news organizations are looking for stories for their annual *Roe v. Wade* coverage. This is a great opportunity to get your message in print and out over the airwaves. Sometimes you can get a news story in advance of an event. We have had stories giving the time and location of rallies, vigils, and other events. This amounts to free advertising and also lets the community know there are people out there who care enough about babies to stand up for them.

If there is a big abortion vote scheduled in Congress, drop a press release with a statement in support of a pro-life vote, tying the need for the bill to your local abortionist. If a poll comes out showing increasing support for the pro-life position, issue a statement with local illustrations of that increased support. If abortion stats show a drop in abortions in your state, issue a press release taking at least partial responsibility by listing all your group has done to decrease abortions, such as helping pregnant women, doing sidewalk counseling, supporting legislation, and so forth.

Understand the audience with whom you are communicating. The reporters are probably not Christians or pro-life. They are busy professionals looking for something unique and newsworthy. Just as you would speak to a child in different terms than an adult, remember to speak to those in the secular media in terms they can understand.

For example, quoting Bible verses at length will not communicate the same thing to a secular news reporter as it would to a Christian church congregation. Churchgoers will understand where you are coming from with the verses, but a secular reporter could find it irrelevant to the story, or even offensive. Also, avoid insider terms, such as "abortuary," as it may make you appear ignorant to a liberal reporter who has never heard the word. Since the goal is to get a message out to the public, it is usually better to state your message in plain, professional language that everyone can understand no matter what their background or worldview is. If leaving Bible verses out of a press release is worrisome to you, consider making it a point to share your faith with the reporter once you get the interview.

Press releases should be short, no longer than four hundred words. This increases the chances that your release will be read, but also keeps the costs down. Most press release distribution services increase the price for releases longer than four hundred words. Be succinct and clever, and above all, sound intelligent. Don't sound too preachy. Reporters may not take you seriously.

Put your main point in the first paragraph. If your release is about a local event, list the date, time, place, and reason for the event by paragraph two or three.

Give yourself a quote. The quote is where you can appropriately use the pro-life rhetoric with abandon. That gives reporters something to use in their stories without having to take time to call you, especially if they are on a deadline.

Put your rhetoric in quotes and the bald facts in the body. Here is an example from one of our recent press releases:

> Overland Park, Kansas—Johnson County District Attorney Steve Howe continues to bungle a massive criminal case against Planned Parenthood—already wracked with scandal—by persuading a judge to dismiss 26 criminal counts related to illegal late-term abortions based on Planned Parenthood's theory that the statute of limitations had run out before the charges were filed in 2007.
>
> "Based on Howe's actions in this case, his political alliances with those who tried to subvert the case in previous administrations, and his over-willingness to adopt Planned Parenthood's legal strategies, we strongly believe that Howe is working in cahoots with Planned Parenthood and is intentionally throwing the case one piece at a time. Because of his apparent corruption, we call on Howe to resign from office. We also demand that a special independent prosecutor be appointed to continue the prosecution of Planned Parenthood," said Troy Newman, President of Operation Rescue.

Notice how the first paragraph explains the issue: A district attorney asked for charges against an abortion clinic to be dropped. If one never read further, he would still understand what we are commenting on.

The second paragraph contains our rhetoric indicating a suspicion of corruption and our solution to the problem. A national pro-life group calling for the DA's resignation and the appointment of a special prosecutor makes the story newsworthy.

If you want your release to go to a wide or national audience, we recommend using a distribution service such as iTrust News, Christian Newswire, or PR Newswire. There is a charge for these services, but your press release will be seen by more news agencies.

There are mainstream news reporters who are open to the pro-life message and will report on it. When you find reporters like that, collect their contact information and send your releases directly to them.

If you are simply putting out a local release that will have little national interest, you can save money by assembling your own list of media contacts. Check the websites of all the newspapers and television and radio stations in your area. Make an Excel file that includes e-mails and fax lines that accept press releases. E-mail works best these days and is the fastest way to communicate, but if you send a fax, make sure your release fits on one sheet of paper.

Don't forget to include a contact name and phone number in a prominent position on the release. The whole point is to have those in the media call you for a more detailed interview. If they can't find your contact number, you may have just wasted your time and money.

Even if you do not get any response from your first press release, keep dropping them. Eventually, reporters will look to you as the go-to person in your area for comments on abortion-related stories and will soon begin to call you when abortion-related news breaks, whether you publish a release or not. This gives you a voice in the community that can alter public opinion and speed the day your community is abortion-free.

RULES FOR WRITING AN EFFECTIVE PRESS RELEASE:

- Limit your word count to four hundred or fewer.
- Put your contact information up front.
- Put your main point in the first paragraph.
- Give yourself a quote.
- Try to come up with pithy headlines that pique attention.
- Use terms that the secular media will understand.

33

FRIENDLY MEDIA AND THE SOCIAL NETWORKING MACHINE

There can be no higher law in journalism than to tell the truth and to shame the devil.

—**WALTER LIPPMANN, AMERICAN JOURNALIST, 1889–1974**

Before the Internet, communication was difficult. In order to publish a press release, I remember typing it up on an electric typewriter, running down to the copy store for duplicates, then placing each release in an envelope that had been laboriously hand-addressed to each news station and paper in our area, before finally dropping the letters at the local post office. How excited I was to own my first computer and dot matrix printer! Later, the fax machine would revolutionize our ability to communicate with the media.

Looking back, it's hard to understand how we ever got along without the latest blazing-fast computer, and a smartphone with an even faster Internet connection. Today, I doubt I would give up my iPhone for anything! With it, I can stay in nearly constant personal communication with our supporters and the media alike.

No matter how well written a press release might be, some

secular news groups simply will not give the pro-life message a platform, unless it is in a story they can use to vilify the movement. Get around their noncoverage by seeking out friendly media and engaging in social networking.

We see a dramatic difference in the number of views a story will receive that we publish just on OperationRescue.org as opposed to stories we both post and promote via press releases, e-mails, and social networking sites.

When we first launched OperationRescue.org back in the mid-1990s, none of us really had any idea about how a website even functioned. We were content to just have a tiny foothold on the Internet. However, as times changed and Americans have become more dependent on the Internet for daily information and news, we had to change too.

In 2004, we completely redesigned our website from a static web page to an active blog and put Cheryl in charge of it. She began to use our e-mail service to publish breaking news and articles that were posted at OperationRescue.org. This drove more traffic to our website and increased our Internet footprint. Soon other sites began to publish our stories and link back to our site. We found that our news was reaching an ever-expanding audience even without the aid of the mainstream media.

Since the advent of the Information Age, many news sources have sprung up that directly cater to pro-life supporters. LifeNews.com and LifeSiteNews.com are both excellent sources of news from a pro-life perspective. They primarily cover all issues related to life, including abortion, euthanasia, embryonic stem cell research, health care, and more. These news services provide free news sent directly to your in-box. Every pro-life supporter should subscribe to them.

These services are scouting for pro-life news and are more likely to pick up your story, so make sure they are on your press release distribution list. Don't forget to include blogs such as JillStanek.com and ProLifeBlogs.com. Do a Google search for additional sites.

Other organizations that cover pro-life stories on a national level include Family News in Focus (a service of Focus on the Family), World News Group (publisher of *World* magazine), and One-NewsNow (the American Family Association). A simple Google search can help you identify others.

There are many more kinds of friendly media that can help you as well. WorldNetDaily, or WND, is a prime example. We consider having a story on WND.com like "hitting the jackpot." It is one of the most widely read websites on the Internet, and its stories are routinely picked up by the Drudge Report, which has national influence over the news. WND writers are particularly interested in publishing evidence of botched abortions, but if you submit your photos and story to them, it should be done quickly to keep the story fresh and exclusive. WND will also publish hot, breaking news, especially if it involves a violation or denial of constitutional rights to free speech and assembly, such as an unjust arrest, police beating peaceful pro-lifers, government intimidation of pro-life activists, and so forth.

Don't neglect your local Christian media. Submit your releases, stories, and editorials to Christian newspapers and radio stations. This will not only help to educate the church, but may help you recruit new activists to the cause.

Operation Rescue is also interested in publishing stories, especially related to evidence of abortion abuses. Stories posted on our website and released by us tend to garner more national attention, especially friendly media, than if a story is published by a local group. We will also publish documentation of abuses on AbortionDocs.org, where the information is available to anyone with an Internet connection.

Track your progress using an analytics programs, such as Google Analytics. Most websites and e-mail distribution services provide statistics that help you see what messages are popular and which ones are not. You should periodically take time to evaluate your web stats, open rates, page views, and the like. It will also help you understand which areas of communication are working and which are less successful. Such evaluations can help you identify and jettison the "millstones" while streamlining your communications for greater efficiency.

In the past few years, social networking sites have exploded onto the Internet and have become a major means of communication and news for the average person. Those who resist plunging into the world of social networking are passing up an amazing opportunity to communicate with large numbers of people instantly and for free. If a thirteen-year-old can figure it out, you can too.

Since we first began to communicate on the Internet, we have expanded our Web presence to include social networking accounts. Facebook pages, Twitter feeds, YouTube channels, and the like promote the message of Operation Rescue to exponentially more people around the globe than we could ever reach without them. It is not unusual to get more views on our Facebook page or YouTube channel in a day than we get to our main website.

To make the most of a social networking account, you should have a smartphone. This will allow you to post anytime, anywhere, especially as news or events are breaking. There are apps—many free—that can make managing your social networking accounts easy. We recommend the iPhone because it works so well and has an amazing array of apps that can help you edit and post photos and videos, schedule your status updates, and make you look amazingly professional and tech savvy, even if you are not. The iPhone models 4s and higher have a better-than-average camera that takes great photos and video. These files can be texted, e-mailed, or posted to social networking sites right from the phone. It alleviates the worry of those who are not tech savvy of how to get a picture off the cell phone, which on older cell phones can be a bit complicated.

It seems as if everyone today has a Facebook account. The social networking site boasts of 1.2 billion active users worldwide. If your organization doesn't already have one, set up a group page on Facebook and post to it every day. Of course, your press releases should post there, but you should be creative. Posting provocative comments or questions can stir a huge conversation about the sanctity of life and help influence those in your circle to be more proactive on life issues.

Pictures are particularly popular on Facebook and other social networking sites. Post them regularly. Smartphone apps such as Instagram can broadcast your photos even further with greater visibility.

Images known as "memes" are also extremely popular and draw attention to your message in a very effective way. A *meme* is an image that usually contains a message. The wittier it is, the better. You can use photo-editing software such as Photoshop to generate your own memes. If you don't have that kind of software, there are sites on the Internet that help you easily make and share memes. Just Google "meme generator" to choose from several available. There are also smartphone apps that do the same thing.

It's good to put your website address on the meme and post it to as many social networking sites as possible. As the meme is passed around, more people will be exposed to your organization, group, or blog. This will help increase your influence and effectiveness.

Twitter.com is a microblogging site that allows anyone with a free account to post in 140 characters or less. It's fast and easy. The brevity of tweets makes it a cinch for people to quickly breeze through their Twitter feeds and pick up on comments, news, or articles that are of interest, while ignoring those that are not.

Most news stories and websites have "share" buttons that allow you to quickly post a story to Twitter, Facebook, or other social networking sites. We love using that to share our stories with our followers and forward links of news stories that advance the pro-life cause.

Sign up for YouTube and post videos that you take or create. You never know when a video will "go viral" and become the talk of the Internet.

We take audio files of 911 calls, create short videos, and post them on YouTube. One video published in July 2011 featured a 911 call from Southwestern Women's Options, a late-term abortion clinic in Albuquerque, New Mexico. It was titled, "911 Call Botched Late Term Abortion on 17-Year Old." As of this writing, it has well over 300,000 views and continued to be viewed by four to six hundred people every day over a year after it was published. Eighty-five percent of the viewers are women, which means this one video is continuing to educate hundreds of women per day about the dangers of abortion, without our having to lift a finger. This makes YouTube a "must-have" social networking site in your toolbox for getting the pro-life message out.

Join as many social networking sites as you can manage, but remember to maintain them by posting to them as often as possible. The more you post, the greater influence you will have. This will amplify your voice and help you make a real difference in the lives of real people.

By effectively using friendly media and the social networking machine, it is possible to bypass the obstructionists in the mainstream media and become ever more effective at spreading the pro-life message so as to stop the killing once and for all.

WHAT'S A MEME?

An Internet meme is usually a photo or image that expresses an idea in a clever or creative way and helps it rapidly spread through sharing, usually on social networking sites. Memes are great ways to share pro-life teachings or viewpoints. A meme can be as simple as a background with text or a complex Photoshop masterpiece. The more creative or powerful the content of the meme, the greater the chances it will be widely shared. When producing memes, always include your website. That will increase your message's visibility, which, after all, is the purpose of a meme in the first place!

34

STRATEGIC PROTESTS

Never be afraid to raise your voice for honesty and truth and compassion against injustice and lying and greed. If people all over the world . . . would do this, it would change the earth.

—**WILLIAM FAULKNER**

The right to protest is a precious American constitutional right guaranteed by the First Amendment. Everyone in this nation has the God-given right to walk out onto the public sidewalk and voice an opinion on the issue of his or her choice.

Protests just for the sake of educating the general public are awesome, but lately, as we have had to more carefully consider the best way to use our time and resources for optimum impact, the strategic protest has become a preferred tactic.

The strategic protest can be used like the exclamation point at the end of a sentence, or to send the message that we will not go quietly into the night as long as babies are dying.

When twenty-three-year-old Magdalena Ortega-Rodriguez was literally butchered to death during a botched abortion attempt by abortionist Suresh Gandotra in San Ysidro, California, we sprang into gear with press releases and calls for action to everyone from the medical board to the district attorney. It was a horrific case. Magdalena bled to death from severe pelvic lacerations received during an incomplete abortion at a run-down strip mall clinic just across the border from Mexico. An emergency room nurse told reporters she had never seen anything like it, and hoped she never would again.

We held an event that was part protest and part candlelight vigil. Surrounded by news cameras and reporters, we lit candles for Magdalena and her baby and held signs denouncing abortion. We gave the community the image of caring people praying for Magdalena's family and calling for answers.

This served to focus on Magdalena and her baby as the victims and on Gandotra as the victimizer. Because of this case, the medical board was prompted to act on two previous complaints that had become lost in the bureaucratic tangle of apathy and red tape. Gandotra was forced to surrender his medical license. The case, thanks to publicity and public pressure, caught the eye of the district attorney, who eventually charged Gandotra with murder in the death of Magdalena Ortega-Rodriguez. Gandotra fled the country. Eighteen years later, there is still an active arrest warrant out for him in San Diego County that guarantees Gandotra will not be returning to US soil to inflict his grisly brand of incompetence on unsuspecting women.

Pick and choose your battles. Daily protests, while useful outside an abortion clinic, lose their sting and newsworthiness elsewhere. We still remember the hired union protestors who picketed local independent produce markets in suburban San Diego for years. Everyone got used to them and, after a while, simply ignored them. That is the worst thing that can happen to a street protester.

When public pressure is necessary, punctuate it with a protest. That lets everyone involved understand that many in the community are serious and can prompt action as it did in the tragic case of Magdalena Rodriguez.

Become familiar with your rights. It's best to stay on the public sidewalk, where your free-speech rights are rock-solid. If you want to protest at a park or other setting, you may need a permit. Some communities have ordinances concerning the use of bullhorns or limitations on the size of signs. Just jump through hoops of red tape and obey all community rules. It will avoid hassles later.

Signs are important in relaying your message to the public. People driving by a protest want to know what it is about. We recommend simple signs with black ink on a white background for greater readability. Make your lettering large and legible. The more words on a sign, the harder it is to read. Remember the old saying that "a picture is worth a thousand words." Graphic images of abortion victims are effective and draw attention. While the use of these signs is controversial, we strongly support it because we have experienced firsthand how these signs save lives and change hearts. Use them or not at your own discretion.

You may want to notify the police ahead of time, depending on the situation, and assure them that you understand the law and want to have a peaceful event. That can make your protest run smoothly since the police will be on hand in the event a passerby decides to cause trouble.

Designate an event leader. That person will interface with the police to ensure a free flow of communication and manage the protesters who may not know the ropes. Do not block traffic or pedestrians when protesting. That will draw negative attention and could create a safety hazard, not to mention problems with police. There should also be a media contact person. Choose someone who is articulate and understands the issues involved.

If you decide not to notify the police, keep a cell phone and video camera handy just in case there are problems. The Bible says that a soft answer turns away wrath (Proverbs 15:1 ESV). That is wisdom for the ages, but especially for the street protest. You are not there to argue; you are there to communicate a message.

Post photos and an "after-action" report on your website and social networking pages. That way your protest will live on long after the event and will continue educating and encouraging others to take meaningful action to stop abortion.

When taking to the streets to protest, be well prepared for just about anything to happen. Sometimes planned events run like clockwork. Other times, the event takes on a life of its own. Unpredictability is a constant factor in street protests.

In April 2000, Operation Rescue and the Christian Defense Coalition staged a strategic protest in front of the US Supreme Court, which was set to hear oral arguments in the first of two partial-birth abortion ban cases to reach the nation's highest court. For seventy-two straight hours before the hearing, our sleep-deprived group fasted and held vigil outside the court on the public sidewalk, with huge signs bearing depictions of grisly partial-birth abortions. Some even slept on the sidewalk throughout the night watches in order to keep our signs continuously on display. One of our signs towered well over six feet above the sidewalk. Others stretched horizontally for perhaps a foot or two longer, bearing panels with diagrams of each step of the horrific abortion process.

We had sought permits for the event but had been assured that, as long as we remained on the public sidewalk, no permits were necessary.

On the day of the hearing, our numbers swelled. The sidewalk became nearly impassible as reporters and pro-abortion protesters joined the growing crowd, eager to have their voices heard on such a momentous day.

Then the rains began.

Umbrellas were the most precious commodity that morning as we huddled shivering behind our signs, praying for a favorable outcome. Cheryl made a comical sight adorned in a large black trash bag with openings cut for her head and arms.

Just as the sidewalk drama was reaching a crescendo, a Supreme Court police officer instructed us that we were in violation of Building Regulation 6. In all the long and storied history of the United States Supreme Court, there had been only five regulations ever—until that day. Regulation 6, which was created and signed just minutes earlier, limited the size of signs displayed on the public sidewalk around the Supreme Court building to a four-foot square. Of course, our huge and very graphic signs, which before needed no permit, were now in violation of the law and subjected us to possible arrest.

It was outrageous. Now, instead of looking for the quickest way to get out of the rain and into a nice, cozy restaurant where we could comfortably break our seventy-two-hour fast, we were indignant and ready to stand there with our newly illegal signs until the cows came home.

As the eye of the national media watched, one by one, twenty-two of us were arrested, handcuffed, and marched up the steps of the Supreme Court for all to see, then escorted to paddy wagons waiting in the driveway on the back side of the building. The arrests done in such a slow and public way made a huge statement, drawing even more attention to the message on our outlawed signage. In the end, we really could not have planned it better.

Once we got to a DC holding jail, we were split up. Women went into one cell, men into another. Among police, there was mass confusion. The arrests were made by the Supreme Court police, who then asked the DC Metro police to process us. The Metro cops, never having heard of "Regulation 6," were unwilling to help. It was all too irregular. The Supreme Court police had little experience with mass arrests and had no idea how to manage the paperwork. It took hours. Finally, just before midnight, after over twelve hours in custody, there was a shift change and the supervisor on duty ordered that we all be released.

Our nation has a grand history of civil disobedience from the days of the antislavery movement to the civil rights movement of the 1960s to the pro-life "rescue" movement of the late 1980s and early 1990s. Even the Bible illustrates examples of peaceful civil disobedience, including the stories of Rahab the harlot, who hid the Hebrew spies, and the apostle Peter, who boldly declared, "We ought to obey God rather than men" (Acts 5:29 KJV).

In fact, it was the rescue movement that birthed Operation Rescue, which grabbed headlines in those early days with mass arrests during peaceful sit-ins at abortion clinics. We remain proud of that past even though our tactics have since changed as circumstances in our nation have evolved.

Washington, DC, is a great place for protesting, especially if the plan includes peaceful civil disobedience. It is a high-visibility location with plenty of media on the hunt for the latest story. The District also has a "post and forfeit" policy that allows those arrested during protests to pay a hundred dollars for release from jail. Paying that fine completely settles the case and replaces the need to return for court hearings. It's a huge convenience that can help you use the strategic protest effectively to keep the crucial matter of abortion in the public eye at the national level.

THINGS YOU NEED FOR ON-SITE PROTESTS

- Clearly worded signs that quickly convey your message to passersby.
- Pro-life literature to hand to passersby or abortion-bound moms.
- A camera to record or document incidents.
- Ample gas in your vehicle to give a woman a ride home or to a local pregnancy resource center if necessary.
- A cell phone in the event of an emergency.
- Bottled water and sunscreen, especially if the weather is hot.
- Proper permits if sound amplification devices are used.

35

THE WEAKEST LINK

Every society gets the kind of criminal it deserves. What is equally true is that every community gets the kind of law enforcement it insists on.

—**ROBERT F. KENNEDY**

The pro-life movement has traditionally been great at passing pro-life legislation, especially since the midterm elections of 2010, when a flood of pro-life state legislators unseated pro-abortion opponents. In the following years, pro-life bills flooded state legislatures in unprecedented numbers, creating clinic licensing standards, informed consent laws, the mandatory offering of ultrasound images to pregnant moms, late-term abortion bans, and efforts to defund abortion providers.

Regulatory laws are not meant to be a means of ending abortion, nor are they the ultimate goal of the pro-life movement. They are stopgap measures that provide a means of saving as many babies as possible until abortion can be abolished in America.

Some laws, such as the federal Born-Alive Infants Protection Act of 2002, were supposed to ensure that babies born alive after failed abortions receive immediate medical care. However, that law has no enforcement clause whatsoever. There is no penalty, either criminal or civil, for intentionally withholding medical care from tiny infants for the purpose of hastening their deaths. Even when outright murder of newborns takes place inside an abortion clinic, there can be no penalty imposed under the Born-Alive Infants Protection Act.

Belkis Gonzalez worked for an abortion clinic where Pierre Renelique conducted abortions, some very late into pregnancy. It was a seedy storefront abortion clinic meant to attract poor women of color who would be less likely to report if something went wrong and, sure enough, one day something went terribly wrong.

It is a case so bizarre that the most creative Hollywood screenwriter would be hard put to make it up. A baby born alive at an abortion clinic was dumped in a biohazard bag and tossed onto the clinic roof to decompose in the hot Florida sun.

It began on July 19, 2006, when eighteen-year-old Sycloria Williams sought out the services of abortionist Pierre Renelique at his North Miami abortion clinic. She was twenty-three weeks pregnant.

Renelique inserted laminaria, gave her a drug that would stimulate uterine contractions, and sent her home with instructions to return to A Gyn Diagnostics in Hialeah the following morning, when he would complete her abortion.

When Williams arrived at the Hialeah clinic at nine the next morning, she was already experiencing cramping, but Renelique was nowhere to be found. Clinic co-owner Belkis Gonzalez, a woman with no medical training, directed Williams to wait in the clinic's recovery room, where she was given additional medication. As the minutes and hours ticked by, Williams began feeling worse. She suffered the pain of severe contractions and nausea. Her complaints were met by stern orders for her to sit down and keep her legs shut, even though Williams instinctively knew that her baby was coming. Williams was told that Renelique would be there by 2:00 p.m., but as the hours passed, Renelique still was not responding to the clinic's pages. At that point, Williams lifted herself out of the recliner and birthed a baby girl.

The tiny baby was writhing, her chest rising and falling as she struggled for her first breaths. At that point, pandemonium broke out inside the clinic. Gonzalez grabbed a pair of orange-handled desk scissors and severed the baby's umbilical cord, but did not clamp it. She shoved the baby into a red biohazard bag along with caustic chemicals meant to speed decomposition, and tossed the body onto the roof of the clinic.

When Renelique arrived at the clinic at 3:00 p.m., he finally attended to Williams. At a hearing of the Florida medical board held in February 2009, Renelique told the board that he was so confused and unaware of Williams's condition that he started an abortion procedure on the sedated woman even though she had delivered her baby an hour earlier.

"That's when one of the employees came to me and said, 'Dr. Renelique, what are you looking for?' I said, 'I'm looking for a fetus.' And she said, 'What fetus?'" Renelique said (Christine Armario, "Fla. doctor loses license after botched abortion," NBC News, February 6, 2009, http://www.foxnews.com/printer_friendly_wires/2009Feb06/0,4675,BotchedAbortion,00.html).

Renelique and his associates then falsified the patient's charts to indicate that he had conducted the abortion and discharged her at 12:05 p.m. even though Williams did not give birth until 2:00 p.m. and Renelique did not arrive at the clinic until after 3:00 p.m.

An informant sneaked out to a nearby pay phone and called the police to report the murder of baby Shanice Osbourne, as her mother would later name her. The police arrived and searched the clinic but could not find the baby. On second search, Shanice's body was found. The abortion clinic was closed by the state.

Renelique would soon face revocation of his medical license, but never criminal charges. However, because of Gonzalez's brazen actions that directly led to the baby's death, we expected something more.

Operation Rescue publicized the incident and demanded criminal charges against Gonzalez and Renelique. In January 2009, a pro-life legal group, the Thomas More Society, filed suit on behalf of Williams, detailing her horrific ordeal and the trauma of witnessing the murder of her daughter. That lawsuit generated additional publicity and public outrage, and prompted a dramatic chain of events.

On February 6, 2009, the Florida Board of Medicine revoked Renelique's Florida medical license.

On February 20, 2009, forty-four members of the Florida House of Representatives sent a letter to state attorney Katherine Fernandez Rundle, demanding that action be taken to bring Gonzalez to justice for her part in the death of Baby Shanice.

That same day, at the request of Operation Rescue, Rev. Patrick J. Mahoney of the Washington, DC–based Christian Defense Coalition held a news conference outside Rundle's office, demanding action and taking the case to the public. Pro-lifers around the nation began to ring Rundle's phones.

Rundle issued a statement later that afternoon that took on a defensive tone and attempted to justify three years of foot-dragging. "While we understand the emotional perception that this is an 'easy matter,' nothing could be further from the truth," she wrote.

However, public outcry soon prompted action. On March 3, 2009, Gonzalez was finally arrested and charged on two felony counts of unlicensed practice of medicine and evidence tampering. Rundle refused to charge Gonzalez with the murder of baby Shanice because, at twenty-three weeks, there was some question as to viability.

It shouldn't have mattered if Shanice would have lived eight minutes or eighty years. Actions Gonzalez took led to the death of

Shanice Osbourne, and no one denied that. Gonzalez should have been charged with murder.

But even with the lesser charges, Gonzalez faced up to twenty years in prison because she was on probation at the time of her arrest on an earlier charge of practicing medicine without a license.

Operation Rescue sought then to charge Gonzalez with federal crimes under the Born-Alive Infants Protection Act, and was shocked to learn that such charges were simply impossible. State court became our only hope to get justice for baby Shanice.

After almost three years of delay, the charges against Gonzalez were dropped. Witnesses had moved or could not be contacted. Even the civil case was dropped after Sycloria stopped communicating with her attorneys. Belkis Gonzalez got off scot-free. After years of prayer and hard work, the enforcement arm of the government failed us.

Such toothless laws as the Born-Alive Infants Protection Act are, in our opinions, virtually useless. We are thankful that the trend has been toward stiffening penalties for abortionists who break the law. With the successful prosecution in Pennsylvania of Kermit Gosnell, we are beginning to see an uptick in interest in prosecuting abortionists.

But even with all the new laws and their tougher penalties, enforcement has been the weakest link of the pro-life movement. Once the bills are passed, virtually no one checks to make sure that the abortion clinics are following the law. In the past, when violations were discovered, there was reticence on the part of authorities to do their duty in the matter of abortion.

But there are ways to break through.

On the street, many times we have heard well-meaning pro-life protestors, distraught at the carnage of abortion, plead with the police, "They're killing babies in there. Go arrest them!" Obviously, that has never worked. These people are asking the officers to do something they cannot do. With the current status of decriminalized abortion in our country, police would be acting outside the scope of their duties in arresting an abortionist simply because he is performing abortions.

The key is to approach this matter in another way. There are ample laws on the books in most states to close nearly every abortion clinic. It is up to us to figure out how we can use the laws to accomplish our goals. Sometimes the frontal approach works, but more often, it does not.

For years, the federal government tried in vain to prosecute Chicago mobster Al Capone, the architect of the 1929 Saint Valentine's Day Massacre, on murder and racketeering charges. Finally, they began to look at Capone's criminal enterprise in another way. They began to examine his tax filings. In 1931, Capone was convicted of tax evasion and sentenced to eleven years in prison, at that time the longest sentence ever given for that crime. Alcatraz wasn't good for Capone, and due to a preexisting condition, his health deteriorated. Upon his release he was unable to resume his crime wave. Those tax evasion charges, while not what Eliot Ness and his "Untouchables" would have preferred, put a permanent end to Capone's career.

This is where the homework on state laws comes in. Sometimes it's the little things that can close an abortion clinic, or diminish its ability to continue killing babies.

In Redwood City, California, Planned Parenthood applied for a permit to open an abortion clinic. Aided by Life Legal Defense Foundation, pro-life activists sprang into action. The city was ready to approve the plans, but it was discovered that there were not enough parking places at the proposed abortion office location. Planned Parenthood leased extra parking spots from a neighboring car rental business in order to comply with the law. Activists applied public pressure and eventually the car rental company cancelled its agreement with Planned Parenthood. In September 2011, Planned Parenthood gave up and withdrew its permit application. A parking space ordinance and some dedicated activists who knew how to use it had beaten them.

36

OUR SECRET WEAPON—THE COMPLAINT FORM

You will never understand bureaucracies until you understand that for bureaucrats procedure is everything and outcomes are nothing.

—**THOMAS SOWELL**

Once you have identified an area where you believe an abortion clinic is breaking the law, determine what agency has oversight over that area. Some states have a more complicated bureaucracy than others. Your homework on agencies that would have authority over abortion businesses should help you sort this out. As a general rule of thumb, violations pertaining to a particular abortionist, such as a botched abortion or illegal prescribing, would fall under the jurisdiction of the state medical board. Violations pertaining to the running of the clinic, such as illegal dumping or poor sanitary conditions, generally land in the Health Department's "wheelhouse."

Once you determine what laws have been violated and which agency would be responsible for enforcement, it is time to file a complaint. Once a complaint has been properly filed with the appropriate governmental regulatory agency, the complaint takes on a life of its own.

Agencies are required by law to evaluate every complaint. With rare exceptions, complaints must be investigated. Once a regulatory agency starts to investigate, there's no telling what they will discover. Usually, the violations discovered through these investigations are much more serious than what we have originally thought.

Below are two sample medical board complaint forms. You will see that while forms vary from state to state, all tend to request similar information.

DEPARTMENT OF HEALTH AND MENTAL HYGIENE

MARYLAND BOARD OF PHYSICIANS

COMPLAINT FORM

Please complete this form and return to:
Maryland Board of Physicians

1. IDENTIFY THE TYPE OF HEALTH PROVIDER:

Physician	Psychiatrist Assistant
Radiographer	Physician Assistant
Nuclear Medical Technologist	Respiratory Care Practitioner
Radiation Therapist	Radiologist Assistant
Polysomnographic Technologist	Athletic Trainer

2. IDENTIFY THE HEALTH PROVIDER:

Full Name:
Office Address:
Office Telephone: ____-_____-_____

3. PATIENT NAME:

4. IDENTITY OF COMPLAINANT:

If the person making the complaint is not the patient, please provide the following information:

Full Name: ______________________________
Address: ________________________________
Home Telephone: ________-________-________

5. Date patient was treated: _______/________/_______

6. Pharmacy used by patient:__________________________

7. RELATIONSHIP OF COMPLAINANT TO PATIENT:
_______ Patient _______ Spouse _______ Relative
_______ No relation

8. WHAT, IF ANY, ARE YOUR PROFESSIONAL OR PERSONAL RELATIONSHIPS WITH THE HEALTH PROVIDER?

____

9. STATE NAMES, ADDRESSES, AND TELEPHONE NUMBERS OF ALL PERSONS WHO HAVE KNOWLEDGE OF YOUR COMPLAINT, INCLUDING ANY OTHER HEALTH PROVIDERS.

____

10. NATURE OF COMPLAINT: ______________________

12. LIST THE IDENTITY OF ANY PERSONS TO WHOM YOU HAVE MADE A SIMILAR COMPLAINT, INDICATE WHEN THE COMPLAINT WAS MADE.

13. ATTACH COPIES OF ANY REPORTS, BILLS, INVOICES, DOCUMENTS, OR STUDIES SUPPORTING OR RELATING TO YOUR CLAIM. Copies of Supporting Documents Attached:
_______Yes _______No

14. I HEREBY ATTEST THAT THE FOREGOING INFORMATION IS TRUE TO THE BEST OF MY KNOWLEDGE AND BELIEF, AND THAT I AM COMPETENT TO MAKE THESE STATEMENTS.

__________________________ Signature of Complainant

KANSAS STATE BOARD OF HEALING ARTS

COMPLAINT FORM

PLEASE NOTE: Your complaint is very important to the Kansas State Board of Healing Arts ("Board") as it is critical in assisting us protect the public and informs us of any possible violations. The Board will not perform investigations to benefit a personal litigation case or act as your attorney. The Board does not obtain monetary compensation on behalf of an individual or engage in dispute resolution. If you believe you have been damaged or lost money due to a licensed or unlicensed individual, you are free to contact your personal attorney regarding recovery options. Board investigations and reviews are not subject to discovery by private litigants. Only public action will be disclosed to the complainant and/or the public. We only have authority over the individuals we license:

M.D. (Medical Doctor)
P.A. (Physician Assistant)
O.T.A. (Occupational Therapist Assistant)
D.O. (Osteopathic Doctor)
P.T. (Physical Therapist)
R.T. (Respiratory Therapist)
D.C. (Chiropractor)
P.T.A. (Physical Therapy Assistant)
A.T. (Athletic Trainer)
D.P.M. (Podiatrist)
L.R.T. (Radiologic Technologists)
Contact Lens Distributors
N.D. (Naturopathic Doctor)
O.T. (Occupational Therapist)

INSTRUCTIONS:

PRACTITIONER(S) AGAINST WHOM ALLEGATION IS MADE:
Please include the first name, last name, and appropriate title (as listed above):
NAME:
ADDRESS:
PHONE:

PERSON MAKING COMPLAINT:
(Please notify this agency if the following information changes.)
NAME:
ADDRESS:
PHONE:

PATIENT INFORMATION:
NAME:
ADDRESS:
DATE OF BIRTH:
SSN:
PHONE:

FACILITIES INVOLVED IN THE INCIDENT:
(Hospitals, Nursing Homes, Clinics, Etc.)
FACILITY:
ADDRESS:
PHONE:
FACILITY:
ADDRESS:
PHONE:

WITNESS(ES) TO THE INCIDENT:
NAME:
ADDRESS:
PHONE:
NAME:
ADDRESS:
PHONE:

PLEASE LIST A FRIEND OR RELATIVE WHO WILL KNOW YOUR MOST CURRENT ADDRESS AND PHONE NUMBER.
NAME:
ADDRESS:
PHONE:

Please describe in detail all allegations against the practitioner(s). Describe each incident with specific dates and list any witnesses. Attach copies of any documents you have concerning the allegations.

DATE OF INCIDENT:
PATIENT'S NAME:
YOUR RELATIONSHIP TO PATIENT, IF OTHER THAN YOURSELF:

I acknowledge that the Kansas State Board of Healing Arts may provide a copy of this form to the person against whom the allegations are made.

I agree to testify in any hearings which may arise as a result of these allegations. The statements I have made are true and correct to the best of my knowledge and belief.

DATE: ______________________________________
SIGNED: ____________________________________

The benefit to signing a complaint form is that you then become the official complainant. Boards usually must keep you informed of the progress of the case. While details of such investigations are confidential, most agencies or boards will notify the complainant on a regular basis of the status of the case, when a disciplinary petition is filed, or when the case is closed. This aids you in follow-up and keeps you in the loop. It also allows you to submit additional information to the case if something new comes up.

Most complaints are confidential and the abortionist need never know who filed the complaint against him or her. This can be important, especially if you are relying on information from a confidential informant. But be aware: some states, most notably Massachusetts, will forward your complaint to the abortionist for "information purposes." That will be noted on the complaint form. (Always read the fine print.) If it is critical that your identity is kept secret, you may want to look for another person, who is not concerned about confidentiality, to file the complaint. Operation Rescue stands ready to assist in the event anonymity is important to you.

When you are ready to file a complaint, go to the agency's website and download their preprinted complaint forms, if they have them. We are aware of some agencies that simply cannot investigate without a proper form being filed.

When we heard that a woman had died from abortion complications in Wichita on January 13, 2005, we knew the first thing that we had to do was get the information out to the public, even before we discovered that her name was Christin Gilbert.

We dropped a press release informing the public of her death and demanding a full investigation from the Kansas State Board of Healing Arts. Later that day, Cheryl received a phone call from a litigation attorney with the board, asking her to file a formal complaint on one of their official forms. Without that, nothing could be done. Even though the board was aware of the incident, without a formal complaint, by law they could not investigate.

Cheryl immediately filled out the form and faxed it to the litigation attorney. Within a couple of hours she received in return a faxed confirmation of her complaint indicating that an investigation would be conducted. It was time for another press release. The public pressure created by public notice of this investigation even elicited a response from the governor acknowledging the abortion-related death.

The public furor had just begun.

Carefully fill out the complaint form using the most professional language you can muster. In the complaint narrative, list as many factual details as possible. As with press releases, try to avoid pro-life colloquialisms, such as "abortuary" or "death camp." A suspected botched abortion may be more seriously investigated if it is referred to as a "medical emergency."

Statements from witnesses who can support your complaint should also be included. Have each witness write a statement that details exactly what happened and includes his or her contact information. Have the witnesses notarize their statements. This will further let the investigators know that yours is a serious complaint that should be fully investigated. If it is not possible to get a notarized witness statement, at least include names and contact information for any witnesses who would be willing to give an interview to the agency concerning the incident.

Include all your evidence. Put any audio recordings you want considered onto a CD and include it with your complaint. Print copies of photos, either professionally or on your home printer, and attach them to the complaint.

It was the audio files of 911 calls that forced a pro-abortion medical board in New Mexico to file disciplinary charges against late-term abortionist Shelley Sella. As previously mentioned, a woman who had previously had a C-section delivery was induced into labor during a thirty-five-week abortion by Sella, who ignored warnings from both the manufacturer of the labor-inducing drug and the American College of Obstetricians and Gynecologists not to use the drug on women with prior C-sections. The woman suffered a ruptured uterus and was lucky to survive. While in the end the board inexplicably decided not to discipline Sella, the documents and disciplinary hearing transcripts were priceless. Front-page stories ran in Albuquerque, and the case carried national significance, putting the spotlight on late-term abortions as never before. While we remain frustrated by the board's outcome, there was good that came out of the whole affair, proving the importance of including all documentation along with board complaints.

We recommend that you file complaints using overnight delivery. This instills a sense of urgency to your complaint. At the least, send it certified mail. Always request delivery confirmation. It costs only a few cents more and could help deter a pro-abortion zealot from simply trashing your complaint or returning it as "undeliverable." It will also give you a record of exactly when your complaint was received and who received it, in the event there is an attempt to deny that any complaint was filed.

Make sure to follow up on your complaint. While board investigations are secret, as a complainant you have a right to know the status of your complaint and whether any action has been taken. Your follow-up calls can make the difference between your case being moved to the back burner or being put on the fast track. The squeaky wheel gets the oil.

Even if a complaint is dropped, don't give up. Keep filing every time you acquire new documentation. Abortionists have glass feet. Because they are continually violating the law or patient care standards, they exist in a constant state of vulnerability to the scrutiny of regulators. We have never met one who completely complies with the law on all accounts. As long as you continue to draw the attention of overseeing bodies to documented abuses, sooner or later something will stick.

37

GENERATING PUBLIC PRESSURE

Let them know that people are watching.

—**PRO-LIFE ATTORNEY MICHAEL KUMETA**

Generating public pressure on the abortionist, the abortion clinic, or those responsible for enforcement can produce results that may not be otherwise achievable.

One of our California attorneys, Michael Kumeta, gave us amazing advice years ago that has heavily influenced the way we approach the matter of generating public pressure. When discussing the matter of public officials who were inclined to sweep abortion-related cases under the rug, he said, "Make it more painful for them to do the wrong thing than it is to do the right thing. Let them know that people are watching."

Public officials will often place political survival above personal biases. If a public official is going to catch heat for ignoring an abortion case, he may go ahead and investigate and prosecute simply to avoid the fallout he knows he can expect if he fails to act. It is our job to make sure there will be fallout and that the official is fully aware of it!

As previously discussed, a well-timed press release or press conference can generate new stories that apply pressure on those who are needed to act. Abortionists generally detest negative news that puts them and their shady practices in the spotlight. Most of them have too much to hide. Prosecutors and public officials often love the spotlight, but not so much when it concerns a controversial abortion case upon which they are not inclined to act.

Businesses that help abortion clinics stay in business are also concerned about their public image and tend to shy away from the topic of abortion. The polarizing issue is simply bad for business.

When George Tiller's abortion clinic closed in Wichita in 2009, LeRoy Carhart made a big show of announcing plans to keep it open. When the Tiller family shut down that idea with the announcement that the clinic would not reopen, Carhart told reporters he planned to continue late-term abortions at a clinic within twenty-five miles of Wichita.

We conducted a very public launch of an online petition that would be presented to Wesley Medical Center, asking them to deny hospital privileges or a transfer agreement to Carhart. We knew it would be problematic for Carhart to open a clinic without assurances that emergency protocols were in place, especially in light of the large number of abortion emergencies we had documented at Tiller's clinic when Carhart was on duty.

The petition was successful at helping Wesley hear the "heart of the people" on this matter and take action to distance themselves from the unpopular abortion trade.

Just hours after we launched the petition, a member of the hospital's administrative staff contacted me, indicating that he would be willing to issue a statement in agreement with that request.

Wesley released the following press statement:

> Physicians do not conduct elective abortions at Wesley Medical Center.
>
> Leroy Carhart is not on staff at Wesley nor has he requested privileges to practice here. Any physician can start a clinic practice without hospital privileges.
>
> Wesley does not currently have, nor will we have transfer agreements with abortion clinics. Wesley never had a transfer agreement with Dr. George Tiller.
>
> Under Federal Emergency Medical Treatment and Active Labor Act (EMTALA), all Emergency departments are required to screen and treat patients that arrive at the hospital with an emergency condition. Wesley treats over 70,000 people yearly in our ER. Our Women's hospital assists in delivering over 6,000 babies every year. We are proud of our role in supporting life.

Due to public pressure and concern that the matter of abortion would damage their reputation in the community, Wesley Medical Center kicked LeRoy Carhart to the curb.

But the statement actually went further. Wesley Medical Center issued the policy statement that elective abortions would not be done at the hospital, portraying itself as an institution that has a role in "supporting life." Once known as the only local hospital that would take Tiller's abortion patients, Wesley's statement rebranded the hospital as being strongly pro-life.

The Wesley petition and the public pressure it had generated worked like a charm.

The press conference is another effective tool we use to generate public pressure. Press conferences should be scheduled preferably during the morning hours. This is for the convenience of reporters who will have stories to write on a deadline or video packages to produce by news time.

Choose a location that will add to the story and give news camera operators an image that tells the story. In the event of an abortion death, hold a press conference in conjunction with a candlelight vigil outside the abortion clinic that is responsible. A press conference outside a prosecutor's office might be appropriate if you are calling for criminal charges. Medical boards that are slow to act in important cases might be motivated to move a complaint onto the fast track if they see television cameras and reporters outside their office, filming you demanding action.

Capitalize on the press coverage by initiating phone calls and/or e-mail campaigns. No one likes having his or her phone ring off the hook or a barrage of e-mails. The person will either take evasive action or "oil the squeaky wheel."

One Kansas district attorney, who was supposed to be prosecuting Planned Parenthood on a criminal case of over a hundred charges, was the frequent object of e-mails generated by our supporters. As a result, he changed his website and ditched the e-mail address that had been used by district attorneys in that office for years. Soon after, he dropped all charges against Planned Parenthood. He made it very clear that he did not want to hear the public backlash.

Other officials have responded well to public pressure. In Massachusetts, Eileen Smith lost her daughter, Laura, whose story we told earlier, to complications from a negligent abortion inflicted upon her by Rapin Osathanondh. Concerned that criminal wrongdoing had led to her daughter's death, Eileen attempted to contact the district attorney, but her calls went unanswered. She reached out to Operation Rescue for help. We dropped a press release about Laura's tragic death and asked supporters to contact the DA and urge him to file criminal charges. Within hours, that prosecutor contacted Mrs. Smith from his cell phone while attending meetings in another state and arranged to meet with her. As a result, Osathanondh was charged with manslaughter in the death of Laura Hope Smith, convicted, and sentenced to jail.

When you have a hot story, don't allow it to cool off. Keep it in the news. Blog about it. Produce a short video for YouTube, explaining the case. Drop a press statement anytime there are developments. We have used postcard campaigns, petitions, protests, and social networking sites to generate public pressure and compel enforcement. The avenues for keeping a story in the public eye and generating the pressure that can lead to action are nearly unlimited. Think outside the box, and be creative in looking for newsworthy ways to keep the pressure on.

SUGGESTIONS ON HOW TO GENERATE PUBLIC PRESSURE:

- Drop a press release.
- Hold a press conference.
- Circulate an online petition.
- Conduct a phone call or e-mail campaign.
- Conduct a peaceful protest.
- Write a letter to the editor of your local paper.
- Mail postcards around town with information about your issue.
- Put up a billboard.
- Create memes for social networking sites.
- Be creative!

38

THE ABORTION COLLABORATORS

He who passively accepts evil is as much involved in it as he who helps to perpetrate it. He who accepts evil without protesting against it is really cooperating with it.

—**MARTIN LUTHER KING JR.**

We like to look at an abortion business as a stool with three legs. The stool needs the legs' support to continue functioning. Remove a leg, and the stool topples over. It can no longer serve its intended purpose.

Abortionists operate in communities with the support of others. Someone supplies the abortion equipment, services the air-conditioning, fixes the plumbing, picks up the trash, and mows the lawn. Imagine what would happen to an abortion clinic if pharmacies quit filling their prescriptions or the trash company quit picking up their trash. It wouldn't be long before the clinic could no longer function.

That is the basis for the Abortion Collaborators Project. An abortion collaborator is any person or business that provides support or services to an abortion business, usually for profit.

Abortion collaborators have no problem making money from

innocent bloodshed—*as long as no one knows*. For the most part, once their collaboration is exposed, they are more likely to stop their business arrangement with the abortion clinic in order to protect their own companies' reputations in the community.

We have seen vendors enter abortion clinic property with the names of their businesses taped over and their license plates removed. Exposing collaborators like this is a public service. People deserve to know if a local business is in cahoots with the local abortion clinic. The public should be encouraged not to patronize businesses that continue to profit from abortions.

The term *collaborator* is often a negative one. For example, those who collaborated with Nazi Germany during World War II have been harshly judged by history due to the great harm their collaboration caused.

It is time to return the stigma of the collaborator to those who profit in any way from the murder of innocent pre-born children. Exposure of this type is an act of obedience to the scriptural mandate in Ephesians 5:11, "And have no fellowship with the unfruitful works of darkness, but rather expose *them*" (NKJV). Therefore, it is the duty of Christians to expose abortion collaborators. Those who participate in and/or profit from the murder of innocent children must not be allowed to hide their guilt.

In fact, exposure of the abortion collaborator is necessary if there is to be any hope of bringing the collaborator to repentance and ultimately ending the bloodshed. Even those regarded as the vilest of traitors, the Nazi collaborators, were given opportunities in many European nations to make amends for their complicity in treason and murder. The abortion collaborator must also be given an opportunity to repent and denounce any association with the abortion trade.

Spend some time at your local abortion clinic and note which venders come and go. Since you cannot be expected to be at the clinic all the time, ask other sidewalk counselors or activists to help you identify the businesses that work with the abortion clinic.

Photograph company vehicles to document their participation with the abortion business. Documentation is very important, since there is liability to wrongly identifying a business as being an abortion collaborator. Be extra careful to verify before going public with the information. That's why a photo of the business servicing the clinic can be the most vital piece of documentation you can get.

One business we contacted about working for the abortion clinic vehemently denied the business connection—that is, until we sent him a photo in living color of his employees and business vehicle at the abortion clinic. After that, the business severed its ties with the abortion clinic.

Send letters informing the business owners that one of their employees was seen providing services at the abortion clinic, and make a reasonable case for the company to change its policy to exclude abortion businesses in the future. Ask for a meeting or acknowledgment that the company will no longer do business with the abortion clinic. Praise those who agree to stop, and encourage your supporters to do business with those companies.

In Wichita, we published a list of abortion collaborators who did business with George Tiller's late-term abortion clinic. We sent letters to every business on the list, giving them the opportunity to stop supporting the abortion industry and profiting from it. We created a booklet explaining the project and held a press conference to announce our findings. We followed up with the business owners. We protested at the hospital where Tiller had privileges, with signs declaring it an "Abortion Collaborator."

Within a few months, 50 percent of the businesses on our collaborators list had quit. This created problems for the clinic, which struggled to maintain vendors. Trash-removal companies either would not service his clinic, or would pick up only in the middle of the night, when pro-life activists would not see them.

Our Abortion Collaborators project left an indelible impression on the community. Four years after Tiller's abortion business folded, one of his former political lobbyists reopened an abortion clinic in Wichita inside the same building once owned by her former boss. Even after the passage of time, businesses in Wichita were reluctant to do business with an abortion clinic. When the clinic's computers required servicing, she was forced to hire a vendor from more than 180 miles away and pay extra for the mileage.

Used judiciously, the Abortion Collaborators project can knock the metaphorical legs out from under an abortion business, making it difficult to remain in the business of killing innocent babies. Most abortion clinics operate with the support of the community. If you can take that support away, the goal of an abortion-free community is likelier to be achieved.

CONDUCTING AN ABORTION COLLABORATORS CAMPAIGN

- Carefully document local companies that do business with abortion clinics. Take pictures of company vehicles at the clinic whenever possible.
- Before beginning a public campaign, contact the business owners and help them understand that they are enabling abortions. Politely invite them to stop providing services to the abortion clinic.
- Never threaten business owners with protests. For example, refrain from telling them that if they don't quit helping the abortion clinic, their business will be picketed, even if that is your plan.
- When conducting a phone or e-mail campaign, encourage participants to be respectful when voicing concerns to business owners.
- When conducting Abortion Collaborator protests, be sure to include signs with the business name and the term "Abortion Collaborator" or "Abortion Profiteer" or other phrases to that effect so passersby understand your message.
- Give business owners every opportunity to gracefully bow out of their relationship with the abortion clinic; then be sure to thank them when they do.

39

THINK STRATEGICALLY

However beautiful the strategy, you should occasionally look at the results.

—**WINSTON CHURCHILL**

Some pro-life groups believe that an all-or-nothing approach is the way to go. They won't support any legislation—and in some cases will block it—if it doesn't ban abortions outright. We feel that there is plenty we can do right now to promote pro-life legislation that will save lives now while we continue to work toward full abolition. For instance, we can whittle away at the industry by supporting regulations and laws that essentially make it impossible for abortion mills to operate due to their proclivity to function well below accepted medical standards.

This tactic has been amazingly successful in recent years, reducing the number of abortion clinics to all-time lows. With the reduction in abortion facilities has come an impressive 13 percent drop in abortion numbers, according to the Guttmacher Institute's survey published in February 2014.

Think about what kind of laws will get you to your goals, and develop a legislative plan to pass them. We have seen some pro-life groups aimlessly drift through one legislative session after another, enacting whatever happens to be the popular pro-life bill of the moment, with no real plan that will accomplish an abortion-free state. As a result, many states possess a patchwork of laws passed in a haphazard fashion that do not provide the most comprehensive protection for the pre-born that might have been possible with a strategic, long-term plan.

Achieving an abortion-free state is not outside our grasp. Six states—Wyoming, Mississippi, North Dakota, South Dakota, Missouri, and Arkansas—currently have only one operating abortion clinic each. Many additional states have just two or three. The right law at the right time could reduce those numbers to zero. Activists are in the perfect place to help determine what kind of bill might be the most effective at reducing abortions and closing clinics, because we know best what is actually going on at the abortion clinics. We can use that information to help drive legislation.

In response to the Kermit Gosnell scandal in which it was revealed that state oversight agencies had not only neglected to look into Gosnell's "House of Horrors" but had actively worked to insulate it from enforcement, the state of Pennsylvania resumed clinic inspections for the first time in seventeen years. The violations they discovered were staggering! The state also instituted new regulations that require that abortion clinics meet the standards that ambulatory surgical centers are required to meet in order to operate. One abortionist closed his two clinics and retired rather than clean up his clinic to comply with new health and safety standards. In all, nine abortion clinics closed as a result of the new regulations—seven in Pennsylvania and two in Delaware—that were associated with Gosnell.

Laws that restrict abortions provide pro-life activists with new opportunities. We already understand that most abortionists hate regulations and believe they are above the law. Because of that arrogant attitude, we have yet to find an abortion clinic that is in full compliance with the law.

In our work with Fr. Terry Gensemer and the CEC for Life in Alabama, we discovered that the owner of New Woman All Women, a Birmingham abortion clinic that we were working to close, was also the owner of the Jackson Women's Health Organization (JWHO), the last abortion clinic in the state of Mississippi. On January 21, 2012, pro-life activists documented two women being transported from the Birmingham abortion facility to a local hospital. Operation Rescue broke the news and published the 911 recording that indicated clinic staff had overdosed the women.

While I was in Washington, DC, for the *Roe v. Wade* events, I happened to jump in a cab at the same time as Terri Herring, a pro-life lobbyist from Mississippi. Later, Terri and I met up with Father Terry at the Dubliner, a popular gathering spot for pro-lifers near Washington, DC's famous Union Station. Together, we discussed the issue of this particular abortion clinic owner. Terry was discouraged after a personhood amendment in her state suffered a huge defeat just a couple of months before, and she was seeking a new legislative strategy.

I suggested that Mississippi try to pass a law that would mandate that abortionists must have hospital privileges within thirty miles of their clinics. All but one of the abortionists hired by the JWHO flew in from other states to perform abortions in Mississippi. The fly-in abortionists had no local hospital privileges, leaving women in the lurch when it came to emergency complications suffered after the abortionists had left town.

I closely follow abortion legislation and was aware that a similar law had already passed constitutional muster in Missouri. The result was the closure of an abortion clinic in Springfield. A second abortion clinic in Columbia had such difficulty locating abortionists that met the requirements that it was often unable to offer abortions for months at a time and finally gave up providing abortions altogether. That has left just one full-time abortion clinic in the entire state.

Terri took the idea and ran with it. The legislation passed easily and was signed into law by Gov. Phil Bryant in the spring of 2012. The owner of JWHO admitted that her abortionists had been unable to obtain hospital privileges. No one would have them. The last abortion clinic in Mississippi was on the verge of closing. On the day the law went into effect, a federal court judge issued an injunction blocking the law. As of this writing, the case is under litigation. However, we have every confidence, barring unexpected judicial activism, that this law will be upheld. This could make Mississippi the first abortion-free state.

My suggestion was the right strategic plan for Mississippi to create the desired result in the quickest way with the least amount of effort.

There may not be a quick solution to stopping abortion through legislation in your state, especially if you live in a hard-core pro-abortion stronghold like California or New York. Nevertheless, you may be able to pass some laws that work to limit abortion a little at a time. Anything is better than nothing, as far as the lives of innocent children are concerned.

Some states have passed laws limiting state funding for abortions, others mandating that abortion pills be distributed according to FDA protocols. Neither of these pieces of legislation is designed to end abortion, but to limit it to the extent possible. As the nation becomes more and more pro-life—and polling numbers are certainly turning our way—we fully expect to see the election of an increasing number of pro-life legislators. That will make it easier to pass pro-life laws. But even if your state is completely controlled by pro-life legislators, none of that will do much good if you don't have a solid legislative plan.

For more information on pro-life laws and language, we recommend that you consult with a group called Americans United for Life. They are wonderful people who provide solid language for a number of pro-life bills that are designed to pass constitutional muster if challenged. They can help you develop a legislative plan for your state and provide you with tools to help you make that plan a reality.

40

INFORM LAWMAKERS AND PROVIDE SOLUTIONS

You're either part of the solution or you're part of the problem.

—ELDRIDGE CLEAVER

Soon after arriving in Kansas, I was surprised when a state legislator told me that while there was a lot of pro-life sentiment in the legislature, they weren't sure what kind of laws were really necessary. Additionally, they were lacking solid information that supported the need for new pro-life laws. They wanted to help end abortion in Kansas, but they didn't know the best way to go about it. We were glad to make recommendations, provide information and documentation, and occasionally speak in support of legislation, much of which eventually was signed into law.

Legislators depend on people like us to help them understand legislative needs. Even the most staunchly pro-life legislator will need your information, input, and insight about abortion conditions in your area. Dealing with politicians even under the best circumstances can be difficult and frustrating, so be patient.

There is truth to the old adage "You can catch more flies with honey." If you haven't done so already, try to build relationships with pro-life state legislators. If possible, go to the statehouse and have friendly face-to-face visits with them. Let them know you are at their service and will provide whatever documentation they need to support their pro-life legislative efforts.

Feed them useful information and discuss the possibility of legislation to address the particular needs in your area.

In 2005, we documented the abortion death of nineteen-year-old Christin Gilbert from complications to a third-trimester abortion at George Tiller's Wichita abortion clinic. But that was just the tip of the iceberg. Over an eighteen-month period, we photographed more than a dozen medical emergencies that required ambulance transport to a local hospital from that clinic. We took those pictures and sent them to every legislator, urging them to vote for a clinic-licensing bill that was under consideration for the third year. We were told that the bill would pass easily in the House but there was no way to get a two-thirds majority in the Senate, which was needed to override a veto.

We flooded the statehouse with images of Gilbert and of the other women on gurneys being pushed into the emergency room by Tiller himself. We testified at committee hearings. We held an all-woman press conference in the capitol rotunda, attended by several legislators. When the Senate vote came, we got the two-thirds supermajority we needed. Unfortunately, political arm-twisting by the abortion lobby and then governor Kathleen Sebelius produced defectors in the House, and an override attempt failed. However, because we armed our legislators with the information they needed to make a strong case for greater clinic oversight and laid a solid foundation, Kansas finally enacted a clinic licensing law in 2011 after Republicans swept the pro-life obstructionists out of office in the 2010 midterm elections.

Once we identified an issue with our local abortion clinics, we sought out friendly lawmakers who could take our legislative solutions and run with them.

No one expects you to become a legal expert on abortion law, but you can still help provide legislative solutions by helping legislators identify areas of need in your state. Become familiar with national organizations that write pro-life legislation, and keep apprised of what kinds of abortion laws have been successful in other states. As mentioned previously, Americans United for Life (AUL) is an excellent resource, although other groups, including the National Right to Life and the Susan B. Anthony List are also helpful at providing sample pro-life bills.

AUL is a group of attorneys who have carefully studied pro-life legislation and have available pre-written language on almost any subject related to life issues. This language is crafted to withstand legal challenges from the abortion lobby and is offered free to state legislators along with analyses of pro-life legislation around the nation.

In March 2010, Operation Rescue released the results of an investigation into a new process of dispensing abortion pills that we uncovered in Iowa, known as "telemed" or "webcam" abortions. We learned that Planned Parenthood of the Heartland had developed an experimental scheme to allow abortionists to dispense the abortion pill over an Internet video conference system similar to Skype.

Women could report to Planned Parenthood clinics around the state where no physician was present. Each woman would be given an ultrasound examination by a clinic worker (who might or might not have been qualified to perform one), then sit in front of a computer screen for a consultation with an abortionist at another office. The abortionist would then press a button on his computer screen that would release a drawer in the clinic where the woman sat. The drawer would contain two bottles of abortion-inducing pills. She would take one set of pills in the clinic and the second set at home.

This scheme allowed Planned Parenthood to cut corners on

women's health by denying a patient face-to-face access to a physician or a physical examination prior to her abortion to determine if it would even be medically appropriate for her to take the medications, some of which are risk-prone drugs that cause severe and unpredictable uterine contractions. But it saved Planned Parenthood boatloads of money: they no longer had to pay abortionists to travel all over the state. Instead, they could employ fewer abortionists to do more abortions, and make more money for themselves.

Just weeks later, during an appearance of Cecile Richards in Cedar Rapids, a Planned Parenthood official confirmed that the national organization planned to expand the telemed abortion pill distribution scheme to every Planned Parenthood location in the nation within five years. That news caused an uproar within the pro-life community, not just in Iowa, but around the nation. Our plans to pass legislation to ban webcam abortions took on new urgency. Public opinion seemed to favor the passage of the legislation.

We worked with Iowa Right to Life and AUL to craft legislation that would ban the dangerous practice. The legislature took up the webcam matter, and the Iowa Board of Medicine amended its regulations to prohibit the practice. Since then, laws banning webcam abortions have been enacted in at least fourteen states and are being considered in a dozen more. Federal legislation affecting webcam abortions has also been introduced. This legislative action resulted in the scuttling of Planned Parenthood's scheme to expand webcam abortions across the nation.

This is a textbook example of how activism drives legislation. Once the information we had gathered about webcam abortions reached the public, legislation soon followed across the country.

Seeking out language that is already vetted can save you time and heartache. Legislators are usually very grateful to receive prewritten legislation that they know has already been heavily scrutinized by attorneys that specialize in such language. It makes their jobs that much easier.

Because we are not full-time lobbyists, we often refer legislators who contact us to a group like AUL, who work with them to craft legislation that addresses the particular needs of their state. We stay involved by providing documentation and public support as needed.

In Mississippi, we worked behind the scenes getting the documentation we had collected about Mississippi's abortion woes into the hands of state authorities who needed the information to pass and defend certain pro-life laws. Proving the need for new laws is key, and lawmakers need more than just your belief that abortion is bad, no matter how strongly you hold that conviction.

We seek out documentation of abortion abuses in every state and have acquired thousands of documents, with more added to our archives daily. Our website AbortionDocs.org is a repository of such documentation. That database lists every abortion clinic and known abortionist by state and puts all the files we have carefully collected right at your fingertips.

In Kansas, after the clinic licensing law was passed in 2011, it was up to the Kansas Department of Health and Environment to come up with specific regulations and standards that an abortion clinic would have to meet before qualifying to be an abortion clinic. An open hearing was announced, and I was contacted about speaking and presenting information in support of regulations at the hearing. We immediately began compiling documentation of abortion abuses to submit to the department. In all, we assembled twenty-five hundred pages of official records that detailed some of the most shocking conditions and behavior at abortion clinics in Kansas and across the nation. The stack of papers was so big it had to be bound in two volumes.

We each got ten minutes to speak at the hearing, which was split in attendance pretty evenly between pro-life and pro-abortion sides. Among the attendees were abortionists Herbert Hodes and his daughter Traci Nauser, who ran an abortion clinic together in Overland Park.

For some reason, during my remarks, I kept referring to Hodes as "Mr. Nauser." Once I sat down, I realized what I had done. When Hodes addressed the meeting, I was amused when he noted his name and title with emphasis in my direction. He appeared to be put out by my inadvertent confusion of his name. It was humorous to realize that without trying, I had wounded his considerable pride.

Then it was Cheryl's turn. She began to account one horrific abortion story after another, with no gruesome detail spared. The stories went on and on as she methodically worked her way through the twenty-five hundred pages of documents. After about fifteen minutes, she began describing in detail Kermit Gosnell's grisly method of dispatching late-term babies who had the misfortune of being born alive at his squalid West Philadelphia abortion mill. That was just too much for the man who was managing the meeting. He rose and literally shoved Cheryl away from the podium to stop her from reciting the rest of her litany of horrors. In the end, however, the board accepted our reams of documentation and passed every regulation for which we had hoped. Our massive page count had dramatically illustrated the need for abortion clinic licensing and oversight.

41

RELENTLESS FOLLOW-UP

You must be passionate, you must dedicate yourself, and you must be relentless in the pursuit of your goals. If you do, you will be successful.

—**STEVE GARVEY**

Everyone has seen roadside flares that burn brightly for a few minutes, then dim and fizzle out. That could aptly describe many pro-life efforts where follow-up has been neglected or ignored. You need to keep on top of your projects once they are launched and follow them through to the end, even if it is painful to do so. This will send a message that you mean what you say and that you can be counted on to finish what you start. This will give you credibility with your friends and make you appear fearsome to the enemy.

We love it when the abortion crowd describes us as relentless. That shows we have instilled in them the reality that we will never stop until abortion is outlawed or we take our last breaths, whichever comes first.

When complaints are filed, keep tabs on them. If you do not get a letter confirming that your complaint was received within about two weeks, call the agency and ask if they received it. You will have the delivery confirmation receipt, so you will already know the answer to that, but reminding them that you consider your complaint urgent could help expedite matters.

As discussed earlier, follow-up is crucial to open records requests. If you do not get a response on your request and there is no follow-up on your part, you have just wasted the effort you made in the first place.

Be persistent, even when folks are giving you the runaround. One of our dear friends, Tara Shaver, is the Queen of Persistence. She and her husband, Bud, once worked in our office as interns and are now pro-life missionaries in Albuquerque, New Mexico. Tara can be like a dog on a bone. Don't stand in her way when she is trying to accomplish something! We have heard her speak with officials in follow-up to her concerns. She is polite and professional, but she simply won't quit until she gets the answer she needs. *She is relentless.* We should all follow her amazing example of persistence and faithfulness.

For medical board complaints, remember to check the license lookup link on the Internet regularly. By doing this, we have learned of discipline against abortionists whom we have then exposed.

If an investigator calls and asks for additional information, it's best to get it to him or her as soon as possible. We have seen complaints closed for lack of evidence, and it would be tragic to see that happen because there was a delay in getting your information into the investigator's hands or because the task was simply overlooked.

Sometimes making the phone calls to inquire about one of your complaints is tedious or even embarrassing. It is easy to feel like you are being a pest. I know that feeling well. Just understand that your next phone call could be the one that cuts through delay or reveals that an abortionist is set for discipline. You might even get an unexpected piece of information that can guide you in your next move.

When you start projects, finish them. The devil is in the details, so to speak. Don't give the devil the satisfaction of seeing you neglect your work or leave the details undone. Following up is the natural fruit of a long-term goal-oriented vision. People who are working toward something as important as saving the lives of babies from abortion cannot afford to drop the ball. Following up can be the difference between success and failure—and the babies cannot afford for you to fail.

TIPS FOR EFFECTIVE COMPLAINT FOLLOW-UP:

- Keep files with copies of all your complaints.
- Keep a log to record follow-up activity. Include date of contact and the name, phone number or e-mail address, and position of the person with whom you spoke.
- Keep archives of all communications regarding your complaints for future reference.
- Make sure to return calls or correspondence in a timely manner.
- Make notes on a calendar to remind you to check on the progress of a complaint.

42

KEEP YOUR EYES ON THE PRIZE

Therefore, among God's churches we boast about your perseverance and faith in all the persecutions and trials you are enduring.

—**2 THESSALONIANS 1:4**

"Some days you get the bear, and some days the bear gets you." So says a popular American proverb. We have been bear fodder more days than we care to admit, but on the days we get to eat the proverbial bear meat, there is nothing sweeter!

Some days will be good and it will seem that everything is going your way, but you need to brace for the days when everything goes wrong—and it will. Don't be discouraged when your complaints are closed without action or the abortionist wins some minor victory. Just learn from the situation and keep moving forward.

There are a couple of ways to avoid discouragement. First, never put all your eggs in one basket. Plan to approach any given endeavor from multiple directions. That way if one aspect doesn't work out, you can still work your other angles.

Second, always have a plan B for when plan A goes south. A backup plan is essential for success. We have a good friend who is fond of reminding us that if we want to be good at something, we will only be as good as our well-thought-out backup plan. Those without a backup plan tend to give up and quit when their one big effort fails to pan out. Those who anticipate setbacks and already have the next step in mind will keep going and are likelier to succeed.

Our work in Wichita is a testament to the virtues of multiple strategies and backups. When a medical board complaint didn't pan out, we tried a grand jury. When a legislative angle didn't succeed, we moved on to something else.

When George Tiller was finally tried on criminal charges, it seemed that victory was within our grasp. We had put so much effort into getting that far that there was little left in the tank. Wichita was a place where we can honestly say we tried everything within the bounds of the law. There was a real temptation to put all our hopes on that trial, but we knew we didn't dare.

In my mind, it was depressing to think of starting over from square one. Tiller just *had* to get convicted. Of course, that was not to be.

Reporters were surprised to find that after his acquittal (on the weakest of charges, by the way, that could have been brought) we were energized and hopeful, but that was because our backup plan had come through for us. The Kansas Board of Healing Arts had filed that eleven-count disciplinary petition against Tiller based on a complaint Cheryl had filed three years earlier. We were back in business, spinning out all the rhetoric we could and hopeful of victory.

Unfortunately, that came to an abrupt end when Tiller was murdered in May 2009. We never got the chance to savor the ultimate victory of seeing his license revoked or him close his clinic in defeat. However, it wasn't because we were shortsighted or had run out of options. Not by a long stretch. We remain convinced that Tiller would have lost and been forced to close his clinic in disgrace. We were so focused on the task at hand that it was just a matter of time.

Avoid distractions that threaten to divert attention from your work. The story of Nehemiah rebuilding the wall around Jerusalem after the Babylonian captivity is instructive on this point. The wall had been broken down during the Babylonian invasion about seventy years earlier. A city wall served to protect those who lived inside the city from the threat of marauders, invaders, and even wild animals. Without a wall, Jerusalem was a very dangerous place to live. Having a strong city wall was literally a matter of life and death to the people of the city.

There were those who tried to distract Nehemiah with public criticism and personal attacks. Some were outsiders, but the ones who caused the most damage to Nehemiah's work were those who opposed him from within, such as Sanballat and his friends. Nehemiah refused to give in to the temptation of engaging these naysayers on their level or delaying the work because of them. Instead, Nehemiah remained focused and avoided distractions. Because of that, he was able to rebuild the wall and make Jerusalem a safe place for families returning to Israel to live once again.

There are plenty of modern-day Sanballats. Some people won't like your tactics and will let everyone know it. Some may find other things to criticize. Unity is a wonderful thing when you can get it, but if there are those who insist on undermining your work, it may be for the greater good to separate from them and move on. Take the high road. Follow the example of Nehemiah and do not allow them to distract you from the work or from your goals.

We have faced plenty of attacks since we launched our work in Kansas and beyond. When I first arrived in Kansas, there was a tremendous amount of backbiting that had poisoned the well, so to speak, before I even got here. It was all because some of the locals felt that the "kingdom" they had built for themselves was somehow threatened by Operation Rescue in general and me in particular. These people undermined every event we planned. They asked my pastor to force me to stop my pro-life work for at least a year. Some tried to run me out of town with ridiculous, self-serving "prophecies" that were anything but divinely inspired. I would not be honest if I told you none of that hurt. It did.

It would have been easy to allow myself to be consumed by the pettiness and with self-pity, but I knew that I had been brought to Wichita by God for a reason, and I simply could not allow myself to be distracted from that work. When we focused on the work God had put before us and put the naysayers out of our minds, our work prospered in spite of the efforts to destroy it from within and without.

But it isn't just the negative diversions that can sidetrack your work. Often worthy projects unrelated to your objectives can also sidetrack you, so it's important to stay focused. Causes will arise that are no doubt admirable, but if they take your focus and efforts away from your goals, it is best to steer clear of them.

A few years ago we were working a new project to expose abortion collaborators. That project took focus and follow-up. In the midst of establishing it, some well-meaning volunteers wanted to do a pro-life sign wave on a random street corner, with no particular target in mind. While sign outreaches are great, at that point in time that random activity was not going to add anything to the effort to expose abortion collaborators. Rather than conducting an unfocused event that had no real goal except general public education, we could better spend our energies and resources exposing an abortion collaborator. In the end, more than half of the companies that had collaborated with the abortion clinic quit doing business with it. Staying focused helped make that project a success.

We have often seen pro-life ministries branch out into other issues, such as traditional marriage, antipornography, or antigambling. We have avoided doing that because it tends to dilute our message and divert us from our primary goal. Operation Rescue is pro-life, and when people hear our name, abortion is the first thing that comes to mind. No one ever has to wonder what we are about.

Maybe you are a rare individual who can juggle more than one ball at a time. We tried that and have found that it's better to excel at one thing than achieve mediocrity in many. The lives of innocent children need your unwavering defense and your undiluted voice.

43

CELEBRATE

Far better is it to dare mighty things, to win glorious triumphs, even though checkered by failure, than to rank with those poor spirits who neither enjoy nor suffer much, because they live in a gray twilight that knows not victory nor defeat.

—**THEODORE ROOSEVELT**

There is no doubt that if you remain diligent, victories will come. When they do, celebrate them.

Celebrations are important, not to flaunt a success or to grandstand, but to encourage the pro-life community that victory is possible. At the same time, our celebrations serve to demoralize those who support abortion. With the pro-life movement energized by news of success and the opposition discouraged, you create momentum that can lead to more victories that will speed you toward your goal of establishing an abortion-free community, state, and nation.

In San Diego, one abortion clinic seemed to have been around forever. It was by volume the largest abortion clinic in San Diego County. We spent many long days and more than a few evenings over the years praying, protesting, and providing counseling on that long sidewalk that flanked the boxy gray structure. It was a ministry seemingly without end.

One day as Cheryl gathered her supplies from her car to prepare for another long day of sidewalk counseling, Ron Brock, a fellow activist, came running down the sidewalk toward her. Breathless, he described a conversation he'd just had with a representative of the company that managed the property leased by the clinic. Apparently, after fifteen years, the management company had decided that the abortion clinic had to go. They refused to renew the facility's lease and had resolved to boot them out on the street.

We had encouraged the other tenants to lodge complaints about the abortion clinic because they often told us that the clinic drove away their patients. Well, complain they did! The management company told us they were willing to take a loss of income rather than continue with the abortion business in the building. All our years of hard work had paid off!

There was so much local history associated with that building that we had to celebrate. So many abortions had cost the lives of tens of thousands, but many lives were saved as well. Rescuers put their bodies on the line during huge rescues that shut down that part of town and testified to the community in a powerful way that there were those who would lay down their lives to save a baby from abortion. There were years of prayer vigils, Life Chains, and *Roe v. Wade* candlelight vigils. It would have been wrong not to celebrate and give thanks for this victory.

We pulled out all the stops. We planned a weekend of events, including a rally and street event. We invited Joe Scheidler, the "godfather" of the pro-life movement, to come out to San Diego and speak. We gave out framed awards to local activists who faithfully sacrificed to save lives. Everyone had the opportunity to show gratitude to God and to each other. It was a wonderful time that culminated in a barbecue at Cheryl's home and a time of sweet fellowship off the front lines. I still have pictures of that event in my office today. It is a wonderful memory.

Of course in Wichita, when George Tiller's notorious late-term abortion clinic closed after his death, a raucous celebration seemed just wrong. However, we still felt the need to mark the occasion, thank God for His faithfulness, and most important, memorialize the unborn babies who'd lost their lives at that place over the long years it was in operation. After we allowed a respectful time to pass, Rev. Pat Mahoney joined us as we held our somber event.

We visited the sites of all three former abortion clinics that had existed at one time in Wichita and laid flowers to remember the lost lives. We started at the building that local pro-lifers called "the crypt," a bland, gray building on the corner of Pine and Market Streets downtown. Some activists shared memories of peaceful sit-ins and other protests that occurred there during the Summer of Mercy and down through the months until it closed.

Next we visited our headquarters, located in the old Central Family Planning building. We prayerfully commemorated the estimated fifty thousand pre-born babies that died there during its three decades of operation, laying more flowers all in a line under a billboard-sized banner that declared, "The gates of hell did not prevail. Redeemed in the name of the Lord by Operation Rescue."

Pro-abortion protesters took exception to our planned memorial at Tiller's clinic, and some lined the street with hateful signs declaring all pro-lifers to be terrorists. We had no desire for confrontation with those misguided souls, and waited to conduct our memorial on our own terms.

Finally the troop of abortion advocates tired of the vigil and dispersed. We arrived soon after to a peaceful, empty sidewalk. We laid some flowers and prayed on the corner of Kellogg and Bleckley, then moved down to the gate.

At that moment, I looked up and noticed that the signs that for years had identified the long, windowless stucco building as Tiller's Women's Health Care Services had been removed just earlier that day. I was so overcome with a mix of emotions that I dropped to my knees and wept. It was finally over. The most notorious late-term abortion clinic in the United States was closed for good.

It was a bittersweet moment. We had been through what felt like a brutal war in Kansas, and now that war was suddenly over—but not the way we had hoped to end it.

A photo of Pat, Cheryl, Pastor Bubby Hudson who had been so supportive of our efforts, and me with my red, teary eyes hangs in our office in Kansas, testimony to the power of prayer and action submitted under the authority of God.

Whether through a joyful celebration or a somber memorial, be sure to broadcast your successes—even relatively minor ones. Post the good news to your social networking sites, send out e-mails, drop a press release, or hold a press conference. If appropriate, have a get-together or rally and use it as an opportunity to recognize and thank those whose hard work helped bring about success. This will build unity within your team and strengthen them for the work that still lies ahead.

In our national headquarters in Wichita, Kansas, we proudly display our successes in Victory Corner. This is a space in a public area of our office where we exhibit a collection of abortion clinic signs taken as trophies after they closed, as well as photos and news articles of other pro-life victories. We love to show visitors this area and share with them the stories that accompany each sign or photo.

Our office is the ultimate symbol of victory, redemption, and restoration as a former abortion clinic that we bought and closed. We take newspaper clippings of some of our more impressive victories, frame them, and hang them on the walls throughout the office. We display large photos of memorable events that speak to visitors of our purpose and goal to protect every innocent life. We are encouraged every day to be surrounded by the trophies of our successes. They remind us that a final, decisive victory in the abortion war is within our grasp.

But once we celebrate our victories and broadcast our successes, it's time to get back to work. Our goal is clear. We work every day to develop new strategies and tactics that will get us to that goal. We won't stop until we have achieved an end to abortion, but we can't do it alone.

Babies scheduled to die each day are depending on you to be their voice and to work on their behalf to stop abortion in your community. Now you have the tools to get started. Let's meet soon at the "finish line" in Victory Circle and celebrate an abortion-free nation together!

RESOURCES

Below is a sampling of the thousands of pro-life organizations and resources available. You can also find pro-life groups in your area by searching the Internet using the keyword "pro-life" and the name of your community.

PRO-LIFE/PRO-FAMILY ADVOCACY ORGANIZATIONS

There are literally thousands of pro-life organizations—large and small—that are working tirelessly to support and advance the pro-life cause. To locate a local group, search Google using the keywords "pro-life organizations" along with the desired city and state.

OPERATION RESCUE
P.O. Box 782888, Wichita, KS 67278
www.OperationRescue.org
Documents, reports, and exposes abortion abuses while working to end abortion.

40 DAYS FOR LIFE
10908 Courthouse Road, Suite 102229, Fredericksburg, VA 22408
www.40DaysForLife.com
Sponsors prayer vigils at abortion clinics.

AMERICANS UNITED FOR LIFE
655 Fifteenth St NW, Suite 410, Washington, DC 20005
www.AUL.org
Focus on pro-life legislation.

CENTER FOR BIO-ETHICAL REFORM
P.O. Box 219, Lake Forest, CA 92609
www.AbortionNo.org
Graphic images, videos, information.

CHARISMATIC EPISCOPALS FOR LIFE
1472 Tomahawk Road, Birmingham, AL 35214
www.cecforlife.com
Alabama-based pro-life activism.

CHRISTIAN DEFENSE COALITION
P.O. Box 77168, Washington, DC 20013
www.ChristianDefenseCoalition.com
Pro-life/pro-family activism.

CITIZENS FOR A PRO-LIFE SOCIETY
67919 Eight Mile Road, South Lyon, MI 48178
www.ProLifeSociety.com
Working to close Michigan abortion clinics, activism, sidewalk counseling.

CREATED EQUAL
P.O. Box 360502, Columbus, OH 43236
www.CreatedEqual.net
Student outreaches, public awareness.

DEFENDERS OF THE UNBORN
P.O. Box 892, St. Charles, MO 63302-0892
www.stl-defenders.com
St. Louis–based sidewalk counseling and public awareness.

FAITH2ACTION
P.O. Box 33395, North Royalton, OH 44133
www.f2a.org
Pro-family network of activists affecting the culture for Christ.

FAITH AND ACTION IN THE NATION'S CAPITAL
109 Second Street NE, Washington, DC 20002
www.faithandaction.org
Christian missionary outreach to top-level government officials.

FAMILY RESEARCH COUNCIL
801 G Street NW, Washington, DC 20001
www.FRC.org
Pro-life public policy.

LIFE DYNAMICS
P.O. Box 2226, Denton, TX 76202
www.LifeDynamics.com
Working to end abortion.

LIFE EDUCATION AND RESEARCH NETWORK (LEARN)
PO Box 9400, Fayetteville, NC 28311
www.LearnInc.org
Focuses on abortion and the African American community.

LIFE ISSUES INSTITUTE
1821 W. Galbraith Rd., Cincinnati, OH 45239
www.LifeIssues.org
Pro-life educational resource and advocacy group founded by Dr. Jack Willke.

LIVE ACTION
2200 Wilson Blvd., Suite 102, PMB 111, Arlington, VA 22201-3324
www.LiveAction.org
Undercover investigations of Planned Parenthood.

NATIONAL RIGHT TO LIFE
512 Tenth St. NW, Washington, DC 20004
www.NRLC.org
Information and public policy related to life issues. Has state affiliates.

PROJECT DEFENDING LIFE
625 San Mateo Blvd. NE, Albuquerque, NM 87108
www.DefendingLife.org; www.ProLifeWitness.org
Activism, sidewalk counseling in the Albuquerque area.

PRO-LIFE ACTION LEAGUE
6160 N. Cicero Ave., Chicago, IL 60646
www.ProLifeAction.org
Chicago-based activism, sidewalk counseling, training.

PRO-LIFE ACTION MINISTRIES
1163 Payne Ave., St. Paul, MN 55130
www.PLAM.org
National sidewalk counseling groups. Provides training.

PRIESTS FOR LIFE
P.O. Box 141172, Staten Island, NY 10314
www.PriestsForLife.org
Catholic pro-life advocacy and information.

THE RADIANCE FOUNDATION
P.O. Box 4112, Ashburn, VA 20148
www.TheRadianceFoundation.org
Works to educate and activate the African American community.

STAND TRUE
P.O. Box 890, Troy, OH 45373
www.StandTrue.com
Pro-life youth outreach, social networking.

STOP PLANNED PARENTHOOD (STOPP)
c/o American Life League
P.O. Box 1350, Stafford, VA 22555
www.STOPP.org
Information concerning Planned Parenthood.

STUDENTS FOR LIFE IN AMERICA
9255 Center Street, Suite 300, Manassas, VA 20110
www.StudentsForLife.org
Network of college groups working to stop abortion.

THE SURVIVORS OF THE ABORTION HOLOCAUST
P.O. Box 52708, Riverside, CA 92517
www.Survivors.la
Pro-life youth activism and training.

SUSAN B. ANTHONY LIST
1707 L Street NW, Suite 550, Washington, DC 20036
www.SBA-List.org
Supports pro-life candidates, legislation, public policy.

PRO-LIFE LEGAL ORGANIZATIONS

Whether it be the need to protect First Amendment Rights or to file a malpractice suit against an abortion provider, the following pro-life/pro-family legal organizations are there for you:

AMERICAN CENTER FOR LAW AND JUSTICE (ACLJ)
P.O. Box 90555, Washington, DC 20090
www.ACLJ.org
Pro-Life/Pro-Family Constitutional Law

ALLIANCE DEFENDING FREEDOM
15100 N. 90th Street, Scottsdale, AZ 85260
www.AllianceDefendingFreedom.org
Pro-life attorneys with nationwide affiliates
800.835.8523

THE JUSTICE FOUNDATION

7210 Louis Pasteur Drive, Suite 200, San Antonio, TX 78229
www.TXJF.org
Pro-life legal assistance and advocacy. Assists minors whose parents are forcing them to abort.

LIFE LEGAL DEFENSE FOUNDATION

P.O. Box 2105, Napa, CA 94558
www.LLDF.org
Pro-life attorneys, First Amendment defense.

THOMAS MORE SOCIETY

19 S. LaSalle Street, Suite 603, Chicago, IL 60603
www.ThomasMoreSociety.org
National public interest law firm protecting life, marriage, and religious liberty.

PRO-LIFE NEWS/BLOGS

BAPTIST PRESS

www.BPNews.net
News from a Protestant Christian perspective.

CATHOLIC NEWS AGENCY

www.CatholicNewsAgency.com
Covers pro-life/pro-family issues from a Catholic perspective.

CATHOLIC NEWS SERVICE

www.CatholicNews.com
EWTN
www.EWTN.com
Global Catholic television featuring pro-life news.

JILLSTANEK.COM

www.JillStanek.com
Pro-life nurse turned blogger and speaker.

LIFENEWS
www.LifeNews.com
News from a pro-life perspective; free subscriptions.

LIFESITE NEWS
www.LifeSiteNews.com
News from a pro-life perspective; free subscriptions.

LIFETALK VIDEO MAGAZINE
www.LifeTalktv.com
Video newsmagazine from Mark Crutcher, with cohost Troy Newman. Monthly DVD subscription; some episodes available on the web.

ONENEWSNOW (AMERICAN FAMILY NEWS NETWORK)
www.OneNewsNow.com
Internet/radio news from a Christian/pro-life/pro-family perspective.

PRO-LIFE BLOGS

WWW.PROLIFEBLOGS.COM
Pro-life articles from bloggers around the web.

WORLD MAGAZINE
www.WorldMag.com
International news from a Christian perspective; print subscriptions available.

WORLDNETDAILY
www.WND.com
Widely read Internet news from a Christian, conservative perspective.

PRO-LIFE INFORMATIONAL SITES

ABORT73.COM
www.Abort73.com
Pro-life information geared for young people.

THE CASE FOR LIFE
www.CaseForLife.com
Information, including debunking "pro-choice" misconceptions.

THE ENDOWMENT FOR HUMAN DEVELOPMENT
www.EHD.org
Embryonic and fetal imaging.

LIFE TRAINING INSTITUTE
www.ProLifeTraining.com
Learn to make a persuasive pro-life argument.

PRO-LIFE BOOKS/LITERATURE, OTHER MATERIALS FOR PURCHASE

Many pro-life organizations have online stores that offer educational materials, books, pro-life DVDs and CDs, clothing, signs, bumper stickers, and other resources. Check your favorite pro-life group's website. To search for a specific item for purchase, search Google using the keyword "buy pro-life," then the item. Example: "buy pro-life T-shirts."

HERITAGE HOUSE
www.HeritageHouse76.com
Vast array of pro-life materials, fetal models, jewelry, and more.

HUMAN LIFE INTERNATIONAL
www.HLI.org
HLI's store offers a large selection of pro-life literature, books, and other resources on a wide range of life issues.

PRO-LIFE WORLD (STAND TRUE STORE)
www.ProLifeWorld.com
Pro-life resources, clothing, and gear.

PRO-LIFE SIGNS

While every pro-life activist should keep a supply of poster board and markers when signs are needed for specific occasions, a wide range of professionally produced pro-life signs are available for purchase that are sure to make a dramatic impact on the street. Below are our favorite sources for pro-life signs.

CENTER FOR BIO-ETHICAL REFORM STORE

www.AbortionNo.org/shop

Graphic, high-quality signs with images of aborted babies, Genocide Awareness Project signs, other resources. Documented authentic abortion images.

ANTI-ABORTION SIGNS

www.AntiAbortionSigns.com

Large signs featuring aborted baby images as seen in "Face the Truth" tours.

PRO-LIFE ACROSS AMERICA

www.ProLifeAcrossAmerica.org/product-category/prolife-signs-banners/

Non-graphic pro-life signs and banners.

PRO-LIFE SIGNS

www.ProLifeSigns.com

Non-graphic signs, banners, apparel, and other resources.

PREGNANCY CARE CENTERS

There are thousands of pro-life pregnancy care centers, some located in nearly every city across America. Pregnancy care centers can be found easily by performing a simple Google search using the keywords "abortion alternatives" along with the desired city and state. Below are large networks of centers that also can refer you to an office in your area.

BIRTHLINE
www.BirthLine.net
National network of pregnancy care centers.

CARE NET
www.Care-Net.org
Affiliation of pregnancy care centers.

OPTION LINE
www.OptionLine.org
Ability to search for offices in specific communities.

MATERNITY HOMES

Maternity homes provide temporary housing for women during and shortly after pregnancy. Most are faith-based, but some are operated by secular groups. It's good to call ahead to learn about specific services and restrictions before referring a woman for housing. To locate one not mentioned in the Harbor House list, search Google using the keywords "maternity home" along with the desired city and state.

HARBOR HOUSE
www.HarborHouse.org/links/maternityhomes.htm
Links to maternity homes in every state, by city.

HIS NESTING PLACE
www.HisNestingPlace.org
Largest extended pregnancy care facility in the Greater Los Angeles metropolitan area. Accepts older children of pregnant moms for housing. This is one of our favorites!

POSTABORTION HEALING

There is healing and hope for all women who have experienced the pain of abortion. We recommend that women who have experienced abortion and now want to serve in a pro-life ministry go through a postabortion healing program.

PROJECT RACHEL

www.HopeAfterAbortion.com
Searchable database of groups in your area.

RACHEL'S VINEYARD MINISTRIES

www.RachelsVineyard.org
Retreat dates available online.

SILENT NO MORE AWARENESS CAMPAIGN

www.SilentNoMoreAwareness.org
Support for women who have had abortions. Assists those who have experienced postabortion healing and want to publicly speak out about abortion.

ABORTIONIST DISCIPLINARY INFORMATION

ABORTIONDOCS.ORG

www.AbortionDocs.org
Up-to-date searchable database of disciplinary information and other documents related to abortion clinics and abortion providers. Includes a listing of current abortion clinics and known abortionists, recently closed clinics, and worst offenders.

AIM DOCFINDER

www.DocBoard.org/docfinder.html
Contains links to every state's searchable database of licensed physicians and medical boards. Databases often contain disciplinary documents in downloadable PDF format. Others database search pages will supply information on how to obtain documents that are not posted online. We recommend that you bookmark this site!

BUSINESSES THAT SUPPORT PLANNED PARENTHOOD

The list of businesses that support Planned Parenthood is constantly changing due to the success of pro-life boycotts. The organization listed below continuously researches businesses in order to keep the most accurate, up-to-date list possible, and we recommend that you refer to their list when making purchasing decisions.

LIFE DECISIONS INTERNATIONAL

www.FightPP.org
Printed list of corporations that support Planned Parenthood is available for a donation.

ABORTION NETWORKS/ORGANIZATIONS

We recommend that you occasionally check the websites of the following abortion organizations to keep abreast of their latest projects and issues. You may even wish to subscribe to receive their e-mail alerts.

CENTER FOR REPRODUCTIVE RIGHTS

www.ReproductiveRights.org
Legal group that challenges pro-life laws in court.

NARAL PRO-CHOICE AMERICA (FORMERLY NATIONAL ABORTION RIGHTS ACTION LEAGUE)

www.NARAL.org
Abortion advocacy and public policy.

NATIONAL ABORTION FEDERATION (NAF)

www.ProChoice.org
Abortion provider membership and "accreditation." Produces so-called standards and holds conferences for abortionists. Nevertheless, NAF-accredited abortion clinics tend to be among the worst facilities when it comes to clinic cleanliness and patient safety.

PLANNED PARENTHOOD FEDERATION OF AMERICA
www.PlannedParenthood.org
Largest provider of abortions in America. Site has searchable database of every Planned Parenthood office in the nation.

ABORTION STATS

Most, but not all, states have abortion-reporting laws and keep statistics that are published yearly. Many state health departments post reports with these statistics online. These statistics are useful in understanding state abortion trends, the number of abortions in a state, and whether the numbers of abortions are rising or falling. The Centers for Disease Control track national abortion trends, but those numbers depend on voluntary reporting from states, such as California, that have no abortion reporting requirements.

CENTERS FOR DISEASE CONTROL AND PREVENTION
www.cdc.gov/reproductivehealth/Data_Stats/Abortion.htm

ABORTION SURVEILLANCE SYSTEM
Example of state reports:
Kansas Department of Health and Environment
www.KDHEKS.gov/hci/absumm.html

RECOMMENDED READING

ABORTION: QUESTIONS AND ANSWERS
by Dr. and Mrs. J. C. Willke
Reference information that is a great resource for those just starting out in pro-life advocacy.

BLOOD MONEY
by Carol Everett
A look inside the abortion industry and what motivates it.

CLOSED: 99 WAYS TO STOP ABORTION
by Joseph Scheidler
99 practical ideas to be actively pro-life. Available at ProLifeAction.org.

COURAGEOUS: STUDENTS ABOLISHING ABORTION IN THIS LIFETIME
by Kristan Hawkins
Examines how pro-life students are ending abortion. Available at SLFA.org.

GRAND ILLUSIONS: THE LEGACY OF PLANNED PARENTHOOD
by George Grant
History and philosophy of Planned Parenthood.

LIME 5
by Mark Crutcher
Documented abortion abuses that will shock and inform.
Available at LifeDynamics.com.

PRO-LIFE ANSWERS TO PRO-CHOICE ARGUMENTS
by Randy C. Alcorn
Outstanding resource for dismantling pro-choice misconceptions.

RECALL ABORTION
by Janet Moreno
Discusses the harm abortion has caused to women, families, society.
Available at PriestsForLife.org.

THEIR BLOOD CRIES OUT
by Troy Newman with Cheryl Sullenger
Examination of the doctrine of "bloodguilt" and the Christian response to it. Available at OperationRescue.org.

WHY PRO-LIFE?: CARING FOR THE UNBORN AND THEIR MOTHERS
by Randy C. Alcorn
Makes a case for the need for pro-life ministry.

TWELVE THINGS TO DO TO MAKE YOUR COMMUNITY ABORTION-FREE

If you want to create an abortion-free community, it is imperative to:

1. Think strategically and set goals.

2. Become familiar with the abortion laws in your state.

3. Identify your local abortion facility and provider.

4. Learn how to use the Internet to research the background and disciplinary history of your local abortion facility and provider.

5. Carry a camera to document incidents, such as medical emergencies, when out at the local abortion center.

6. Learn how to make requests for 911 records and understand what to do with them once you have them.

7. Use the Freedom of Information Act to make requests for other public information, such as Termination of Pregnancy Reports, autopsy reports, communications between government agencies concerning an abortion facility, and more.

8. Become adept at filling out and filing formal complaints with oversight agencies, such as medical boards and health departments.

9. Effectively use press releases and social media to expose the "dirt" on your local abortion business.

10. Learn how to generate public pressure through exposés, flyers, petitions, protests, etc.

11. Become familiar with friendly lawmakers, and get documentation of abortion abuses into their hands.

12. Relentlessly follow up on complaints and other projects.

INDEX

E

F

G

H

M

N

O

P–Q

R

S

T

U

V

W–X

Y–Z